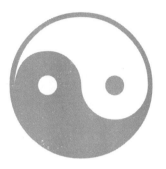

Qigong
for Health
and Well-Being

Qigong
for Health
and Well-Being

FaXiang Hou
and
Mark V. Wiley

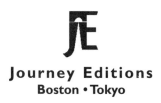

Journey Editions
Boston • Tokyo

DISCLAIMER
Please note that the author and publisher of this book are NOT RESPONSIBLE in any manner whatsoever for any injury that may result from practicing the techniques and/or following the instructions given within. Since the physical activities described herein may be too strenuous in nature for some readers to engage in safely, it is essential that a physician be consulted prior to training.

First published in 1999 by Journey Editions, an imprint of Periplus Editions (HK) Ltd., with editorial offices at 153 Milk Street, Boston, Massachusetts 02109.

Library of Congress Cataloging-in-Publication Data

Hou, FaXiang, 1955–
    Qigong for health and well-being / FaXiang Hou and Mark V. Wiley.
—1st ed.
        p. cm.
    Includes bibliographical references (p.).
    ISBN 1-885203-79-9
    1. Ch'i kung. 2. Health. 3. Exercise. I. Wiley, Mark V.
II. Title.
RA781.8. H675 1999
613.7'1—dc21   98-47042
                                                                          CIP

Distributed by

USA	CANADA	JAPAN	SOUTHEAST ASIA
Tuttle Publishing	Raincoast Books	Tuttle Shokai Ltd	Berkeley Books Pte Ltd
Distribution Center	8680 Cambie Street	1-21-13, Seki	5 Little Road #08-01
Airport Industrial Park	Vancouver, British	Tama-ku, Kawasaki-shi	Singapore 536983
364 Innovation Drive	Columbia	Kanagawa-ken 214-	Tel: (65) 280-1330
North Clarendon, VT	V6P 6M9	0022, Japan	Fax: (65) 280-6290
05759-9436	Tel: (604) 323-7100	Tel: (044) 833-0225	
Tel: (802) 773-8930	Fax: (604) 323-2600	Fax: (044) 822-0413	
Tel: (800) 526-2778			

First edition
05 04 03 02 01 00 99 98 97 1 3 5 7 9 10 8 6 4 2
Printed in the United States of America
Text and cover design by Jill A. Feron

ACKNOWLEDGMENTS

The authors would like to extend their heartfelt thanks to Deborah LeBlanc, Shelly Fleischman, Mary Jane Pullen, Barbara Hornum and Mike Maliszewski for their various contributions and assistance with this project.

TABLE OF CONTENTS

Foreword

Imagine suffering severe migraine headaches for thirty years, in spite of countless trials of various medications. Then, when it seems just hopeless, a stranger from a foreign land figuratively falls through your roof into your living room, administers a few *qigong* treatments, teaches you some exercise practices, and within two months you are headache-free.

It sounds something like a fairy tale, but truth can be far stranger than fiction.

One Saturday in late September, 1991 I found myself in the backseat of a car being driven by a dear friend, a Western medical practitioner who was born in China. We were accompanied by each of our mothers and were traveling to Maryland to be treated by a qigong master for conditions that had not been successfully treated by Western medical practices.

Most who read this probably know more about qigong than I did at that time. I had never heard the word, did not know what it meant, and could not pronounce it.

Once in Maryland, we came upon an attractive young man with a special presence; he spoke no English and conversed briefly with us through our friend and interpreter. With little conversation, he proceeded to treat us. My friend, who had walked in bent over with obvious back pain, walked out with a normal, carefree gait. At the time, I had no knowledge of how special this man was, nor how special his art was, but what I saw with my own eyes convinced me that this was indeed something unique to my experience.

I soon learned that FaXiang Hou was a master of medical qigong and recognized as such by the major Chinese government accrediting agencies. He was trained traditionally by his father, with the lineage of familial training tracing back five generations to a great-great-grandfather who traveled to Tibet to study for twelve years.

FaXiang Hou had come to the United States, from mainland China, to try to learn English and bring to the Western world his treasured family form of qigong, known as *ching loong san dian xue mi gong fa.*

This unique form of medical qigong, practiced only by FaXiang Hou and his brother, has had amazing efficacy, as both a treatment and exercise form, in relieving numerous acute and chronic illnesses.

We were so impressed with what we witnessed that we invited him to New Jersey, where we knew others who would also appreciate his treatment. Master Hou accepted our invitation and stopped in South Jersey for a day, on his way to Chinatown in New York City, where he was scheduled to give a presentation.

The rest became history in a way that was probably unusual at the time. I had worked in a Western medical environment for over thirty-five years and had a husband, two sons, and a brother who were physicians. Perhaps it was my interest in yoga over most of these years that encouraged me to "see what this is about."

In February 1993, I suffered a severe ski injury with MRI-verified complete cruciate tear, ninety percent medial collateral tear, and tibial head fractures, with recommendation for cruciate reconstruction with a cadaver tendon. Since surgery could not be performed for eight weeks, because of the huge swelling of my knee, I opted for treatment by Master Hou and performed the exercises that he taught, as directed. Eight weeks later, I returned to the treating orthopedist for probable surgical scheduling, and was discharged and advised just to swim to further rehabilitate my knee. I have no awareness at this time of prior knee injury and am able to ski, roller blade, hike, and maintain an active lifestyle.

In October, 1996 I was in a very bad motor vehicle accident and struck my jaw. I suffered severe lip laceration, a fractured tooth, immediate severe swelling about the mouth, as well as severe left arm injury with internal bleeding and massive immediate swelling of my arm, hand, and fingers to twice their normal size. With three treatments and within two days following injury, the swelling and pain were at least eighty percent reduced, and I have required no further treatment. My car did not fare so well and took months to repair.

I am pleased to tell of my success with the practice of Master Hou's qigong form and hope that it will inspire others to use this vehicle to help themselves.

In the past six years, I have seen what I consider intriguing results in students and patients suffering from a remarkable variety of illnesses and injuries, too numerous to mention. These include chronic fatigue syndrome, reflex sympathetic dystrophy, collagen diseases, musculoskeletal injuries, heel spurs, hypertension, asthma, digestive problems, AIDS, leukemia, parasitosis, and scleroderma with severe Raynaud's syndrome. I have also seen great success in the treatment of dysfunctional uterine bleeding, amenorrhea, breast masses, and infertility.

As a student, I have learned over time that Master Hou's form can be used as a tool for treating or preventing imbalances in energy flow in your body, which can treat and prevent many "dis-eases." What is required is daily practice for at least twenty minutes a day for at least 100 days. Of course, the more practice time spent, the better results achieved.

For many Westerners, the theoretical concepts of qigong are difficult to comprehend, particularly early on, for many of the terms used are not part of our vocabulary or culture. This book is written with that in mind. It is my experience that with regular practice one's understanding also grows.

If you are willing to open the door and step into the room, you may well discover a method of tuning into and tuning up your body and mind, which carries the power of an ancient discipline with its purity preserved over paternal ancestral lines, with practical modifications that fit very well in our modern society.

I wish you a state of well-being, physical and mental, beyond what you may ever have thought you could achieve, but which I have seen many accomplish with the practice of qigong.

I am grateful to Master Hou for sharing a portion of his legacy with us.

—Rochelle Fleischman

Introduction

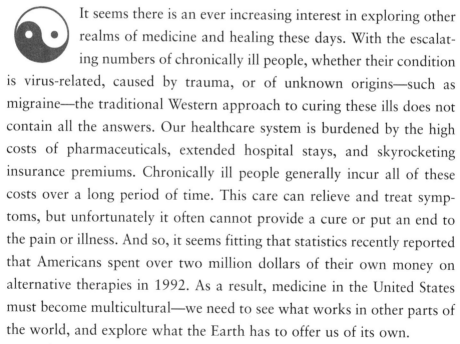It seems there is an ever increasing interest in exploring other realms of medicine and healing these days. With the escalating numbers of chronically ill people, whether their condition is virus-related, caused by trauma, or of unknown origins—such as migraine—the traditional Western approach to curing these ills does not contain all the answers. Our healthcare system is burdened by the high costs of pharmaceuticals, extended hospital stays, and skyrocketing insurance premiums. Chronically ill people generally incur all of these costs over a long period of time. This care can relieve and treat symptoms, but unfortunately it often cannot provide a cure or put an end to the pain or illness. And so, it seems fitting that statistics recently reported that Americans spent over two million dollars of their own money on alternative therapies in 1992. As a result, medicine in the United States must become multicultural—we need to see what works in other parts of the world, and explore what the Earth has to offer us of its own.

Alternative therapies are vast and diverse worldwide, and are beginning to appear in more places throughout the United States. In China, they have been using a medical system that employs the high-tech life-saving Western modes of surgery, pharmaceuticals, and so on, concurrently with the use of acupuncture, special diets to aid healing, herbal remedies, and the practice of *qigong*. Research has shown that improvements in patients' conditions when they are treated with these multiple methods are impressive. Think of where so many athletes, arthritis sufferers, and heart patients would be today without the physical therapies now being used to relieve and rehabilitate them. A short time ago these therapies were unheard of, and chronic pain and discomfort was only relieved temporarily through the use of analgesics. A combined modality of care has provided this step up in treatment. Should we step back to the days of chronic bedside treatment? No. Neither should we shrug off the concepts that Chinese medical theory has to offer in terms of making even more headway in the fight against disease and pain.

Today, in Shanghai and Beijing, scientists are using modern equipment to research and analyze the effects of qigong. They have found qigong particularly beneficial in treating chronic complaints such as hypertension, asthma, arthritis, and headaches, among other ailments. This indicates the seriousness with which modern-day scientists and physicians are considering the existence and importance of *qi* and the practice of qigong today. It is in this light that we wrote this instructional manual.

This book is not meant to be a dissertation on the phenomenon of qi, nor a scholarly presentation on the art of qigong or traditional Chinese medicine. It is, rather, an easy to read and understand instructional book on the fundamental practice of qigong for health and well-being. As a result, we have not included the standard charts on the five elements and meridian systems found in many qigong books (the interested reader is directed to the books listed in the Bibliography). Although the book opens with chapters on Chinese healthcare systems and an overview of the development of the qigong form presented herein, this is meant more as a prelude to help the reader understand where these exercises come from and how they relate to the whole of Chinese medicine.

Our aim in writing this book has been to introduce you to the practice and philosophy of qigong in a positive way, to enable you to reap the benefits of the improved health and vitality that it brings. We have endeavored, through description and illustration, to make the exercises easy to learn and easy to do.

To facilitate this ease, we have divided the book into three parts. Part One, General Background, puts the topic in perspective by outlining the Chinese medical model, which has existed for over 3,000 years, and offers the reader an easily understood definition and description of what qigong is, in theory and practice.

Part Two, Hou Family Qigong, offers the reader a glimpse of Master Hou's life and background in qigong, gives a description of the *ching loong san dian xue mi gong fa qigong* form, and concludes with a number of testimonials to the effectiveness of the system based on his patients' and students' first-hand experiences.

Part Three, Building Foundation Qigong, examines the eight primary qigong points on the body used in the fundamental qigong program that follows. Once the importance and location of these points are understood, the reader is presented with seven foundation exercises to practice, followed by six advanced animal and element exercises. The practice of these exercises for at least 100 days will ensure that the reader moves stagnant energy out of his body, maintains open qi points and free flow of qi throughout the meridian system, and stores special energy. The foundation qigong exercises are illustrated with step-by-step photographs, consisting of thirteen formal exercises.

An interview with Master Hou follows, containing the most commonly asked questions at his seminars and classes. This offers additional insights and supplements the information presented in Parts One and Two.

The book concludes with an Afterword, a Glossary of terms used in the book, and a Bibliography containing books on the subject that we recommend as supplemental reading.

We wish you much luck and happiness on your qigong journey toward health and well-being.   —FaXiang Hou, Mark V. Wiley

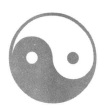

PART ONE
General Background

CHAPTER 1
Traditional Healthcare in China

 ## THE CHINESE MEDICAL MODEL

All human societies have belief systems and practices that people turn to in order to identify disease and effect a cure. Both physical and supernatural explanations for the etiology (or cause) and treatment of illness and disease may be sought at various times for various reasons. Coinciding with the cause of the illness is the patient's or physician's choice of treatment modality. In China, and now around the world, the practice of qigong has become a primary treatment choice.

Traditional Chinese medicine is a system best described as holistic. It is a highly somatic system that depends upon various methodologies in the diagnosis and treatment of illness and disease. Its underpinnings are based upon the view that the human body is a reflection of the natural (physical) world, and that what exists within is a reflection of what is present on the outside. This argues for what might be considered a somatic/psychophysical model of healing. The biological aspect consists of the basic structure of the human body (e.g., muscles, tissues, organs, nerves). The psychophysical principle consists in the belief that a latent intrinsic energy known as qi permeates the body. In the Chinese medical model, it is the relationship between the intrinsic energy and the grosser physical body that determines the degree to which illness or health prevail.

Like other cultures and societies, China has an integrated system of beliefs and practices which, while able to identify and cure illness and disease, exists primarily as a system of preventative medicine. Several different techniques or intervention procedures constitute traditional Chinese systems of healthcare. These include the practice of qigong exercise, and treatment through acupuncture and herbology. The application of such preventative or restorative procedures is determined by the perceived etiology of an illness or disease.

UNDERLYING CULTURAL CONCEPTS

In order to understand how Chinese medical intervention procedures are employed, several concepts unique to traditional Chinese medicine should be discussed. The first set of terms commonly used to describe various opposing physical conditions relating to the body is *yin* and *yang*. Metaphysically speaking, yin and yang are two polar energies that, by their fluctuation and interaction, are the cause of the universe. Yang corresponds to what is masculine, active, creative, bright, and hard. Yin is the feminine, passive, receptive, dark, and soft. As these concepts are applied to medical analysis of the human body, yin refers to the tissues of the organ, while yang refers to its activity. Deficiencies of either of these lead to some type of imbalance. In yin deficiency, the organ does not have enough raw materials to function. In yang deficiency, the organ does not react adequately when needed. Again, these two conditions are connected in a system of interdependence and interrelatedness.

Related to the concept of yin and yang is the system of five elements that emerge out of the interaction of yin and yang. These five elements—water, fire, wood, metal, and earth—do not constitute real substances but rather are viewed as abstract forces and symbols for certain basic characteristics of matter. Historically, these elements not only give rise to each other but can also conquer or destroy one another. This system of five elements is related to the interaction of different organs in the body. The five elements system is based on the view that each organ either nourishes or inhibits the proper functioning of another organ, just as the basic elements also act either adversely or beneficially on each other. Organs may also be divided into two groups of yin and yang organs. The liver, heart, spleen, lungs, and kidney are members of the yin group, because they are viewed as being more substantial or solid in nature. Yang organs are hollow and functional and include the small intestine, stomach, large intestine, and bladder. It should also be understood that synergistic relationships exist among all the different organs. It is an analysis of how these organs interact that assists a traditional Chinese doctor with diagnosing a particular illness or disease and its symptoms.

The relationship of yin and yang within the human body has a great influence on one's health. Perfect harmony between the two primal forces brings good health. The practice of qigong is aimed at achieving this perfect harmony. Qigong exercises harness the flowing of the yin and the yang. Power and strength are brought forth by the practice of qigong.

Another central concept in traditional Chinese medicine is the phenomenon of qi. Generally speaking, qi refers to the vital energy, life force, or cosmic spirit that pervades all things. It is synonymous with primordial energy. In the human body, qi is accumulated in an area two finger's width beneath the navel, called the *dantian* (field of elixir), where it is stored. Wasting of this energy can result in either sickness or death. It is believed that this vital energy or life force can be strengthened through diaphragmatic breathing exercises. This principle is found in such diverse areas as martial arts, Taoist meditation, and traditional Chinese medicine proper. In the latter case, this vital energy flows through the human body along pathways referred to as meridians. Central to traditional Chinese medicine is the belief that one must keep the qi flowing in order to maintain health. It should be pointed out that organs can be accessed in various ways for treatment through specific meridians. Moreover, illness can occur when there is a blockage of qi in these channels. In addition to the fourteen primary meridian channels (which include the *du* and *ren* channels), there are eight collateral channels. These special channels are not connected with the internal organs, as the primary fourteen are believed to be, but are those through which qi flows when there is enough buildup of qi to overflow the twelve regular meridians. Thus, since qi later flows back into the twelve meridians when there is a deficiency of qi in the body, the eight collateral channels serve as regulators for the twelve meridians. Complementing this emphasis on qi and acting as treatments are the earlier-mentioned practices of qigong, acupuncture, and herbology.

ETIOLOGY: THE ORIGINS OF DISHARMONY

Traditional Chinese medicine is spun in a web crafted by Chinese Taoist philosophy and, therefore, does not concern itself with cause and effect. Rather, opposing the Western view of illness and healing, traditional Chinese medicine concerns itself with relationships, with patterns of events, not necessarily with their linear sequence.

Traditional Chinese medicine views cause and effect as one. The traditional Chinese doctor views the human body as a microcosm of nature. The traditional Chinese medical model views the healthy body as maintaining a balance of yin and yang. These two conditions are forever connected in a system of interdependence and interrelatedness. Such a connection finds the qi at once able to move blood and maintain its location; it finds the heart also moving blood and storing *shen* (spirit). When the balance of yin and yang is upset, the body may become susceptible to the harmful effects of a pernicious influence such as dampness, dryness, heat, or cold. It should be noted, however, that in terms of traditional Chinese medicine a pernicious influence is viewed as a natural event. It only becomes a cause of illness when the body reacts adversely to it (e.g., the relationship between the body and the pernicious influence is disturbed). Such a disturbance invariably leads to bodily dysfunction, which can be characterized in terms of the so-called eight parameters. These include external versus internal, hot versus cold, excessive versus deficient, and yin versus yang. A patient's symptoms and physical examination (determined by taking the pulse and examining the tongue), enable the traditional Chinese doctor to recognize a pattern of illness, which, in effect, becomes the diagnosis. After an illness has been given an appropriate diagnosis, a traditional system of Chinese healthcare will be employed to effect a cure. The direct transmission of qi and the performance of specific qigong exercises constitute such a healthcare system.

CHAPTER 2
Qigong in Perspective

QIGONG: A PRACTICAL DEFINITION

Qigong refers to specific health exercises combining Buddhist and Taoist elements. Such exercises are viewed as techniques for regulating the body, the mind, and the breath, and involve movement and self-massage to effect changes in health. More specifically, qigong is the art of exercising the *jing* (essence), *qi* (vital energy), and *shen* (spirit). The nucleus of qigong is the exercise of consciousness and vital energy. The goal of qigong, therefore, is to circulate, build, and balance qi throughout the body to promote physical and mental well-being. As qigong is a cornerstone of the traditional Chinese medical model, it continues to be practiced by thousands throughout much of Asia today.

Qigong is a holistic therapy that exercises the body and mind and increases consciousness. Regular practice of qigong exercises aids in regulating the functions of the central nervous system. Along with exercising and controlling one's mind and body, qigong influences one's physical state in general, while improving one's pathological condition in particular. Concurrently, the practice of qigong evokes latent powers within the human body, enabling the practitioner to use them to their fullest potential. The Chinese believe that qigong practice increases the body's ability to adapt to and defend against the natural/physical environment in which we live.

Specifically, the practice of qigong exercises combines the practice of *xing* (shape-postures), *yi* (intention or concentration), and *qi* (vital energy). To exercise the so-called genuine qi is to exercise the three treasures of the human body (jing, qi, and shen), so as to relieve pain, strengthen the body's constitution, improve intelligence, and prolong life. Traditional Chinese doctors refers to xing, yi, and qi as the "three regulations." Controlling the three regulations through various qigong practices is said to regulate the body's constitution, consciousness, and respiration, respectively. Such regulations are the main principle of the practice of qigong and the primary constituents of the maintenance of good health.

THE VARIETY OF QIGONG FORMS

The varieties of qigong can be divided into four categories containing three areas each. As for a global categorization, there are Buddhist, Taoist, and Confucian qigong practices.

Within these categories, there are three primary applications of qigong. In times past, qigong was used in conjunction with various Chinese martial arts. Practitioners would spend countless time memorizing the so-called deadly points along the meridian system, and the specific time of day and month of the year during which each point was most effective. This was the prelude to using the secret "death touch" techniques, known as *dimak*, to maim or kill an opponent.

The primary use of qigong today is to improve one's health, thus extending life. This is known as medical or healing qigong, of which there are three subdivisions: (1) external therapy, whereby a Chinese doctor projects his own qi into a patient's body to effect a cure, (2) self-training, whereby a person chooses a qigong program and performs the exercises over a period of at least 100 days to improve his or her own health, and (3) a combination of external qigong treatments from a doctor and an individual's qigong training program. Within the self-practice method, exercises are done in any combination of three ways: slow movements, meditation, and breathing exercises.

The third category is the use of qigong for various demonstrative purposes. Many qigong and martial arts masters today use this method for attracting new patients and/or students.

HOW AND WHEN TO PRACTICE

When practicing qigong, one must be sure not to separate one thing from another. The movements/postures, visualization/meditation, and proper breathing must all be done concurrently. It is not the actual movements or shape-postures that are difficult, but the correct performance of them in conjunction with the proper regulation of the breath and the flow of qi.

Proper breathing and control of the breath is perhaps the most important aspect of qigong. Through proper breathing, the organs of the body are strengthened, and their functioning is improved. Inhaling brings nourishment into the body and assists blood circulation and organ function. Exhaling serves to cleanse the body of harmful elements and wastes.

Breath control is necessary for the conduction of the qi. Vital energy is both mental and physical energy. Correct breathing allows the vital energy to flow naturally.

Students frequently ask such questions as "What should we practice?", "When should be practice?", and "How should we practice?" "There is so much to do and yet such little time", they say. And so, the question arises as to whether it is best to do more repetitions of selected exercises or to do fewer repetitions of a number of exercises.

The concept appears very Eastern, and probably very self-apparent to someone raised in an Asian culture. But individuals must simply attune to their bodies, know where trouble may possibly be forming, and exercise, eat, and breathe in a way that will help to prevent discomfort in that organ or area of the body. That is not to say that one can totally prevent discomfort, for discomfort appears, at times, to be part of unblocking a meridian. We learn many exercises and techniques and must choose the appropriate time and way to utilize them. Practice alone will allow you to make such a decision.

Qigong involves sensing our own blockages and imbalances and attuning to the energies around us to normalize such imbalances and maximize energy flow internally and externally, to maximize our health and well-being.

The practices outlined in Part Two will help you to perceive a strong visceral feeling of qi and an enhanced state of health, requiring no special time, place, equipment, age group, or physical condition to perform.

Don't expect too much too soon, however. There will be results if you practice according to the prescribed outline. In essence, you must devote yourself to qigong and make an effort to practice every day, as qi cannot be cultivated by part-time or once-a-week practice. Dedication to practice every day for at least the first 100 days is essential. After the first 100 days, the body has developed the qi and will not lose it any time soon. After this time, the student/patient may practice the individual exercises as needed.

SENSATIONS FELT DURING PRACTICE

During the practice of qigong you may feel various sensations in your body. The most common sensation experienced is an increase of body heat in one of the dantian areas. This occurs as qi is being cultivated and stored in this area. An overwhelming sense of peace and comfort may envelop you as you practice or meditate. This, too, is normal and a positive indication that you are practicing correctly. Other sensations felt include a tingling sensation on the skin and an increase of saliva. Again, both are positive results of proper qigong practice.

Some uncomfortable sensations that the novice practitioner may experience during initial qigong practice include a general heaviness due to incorrect breathing, dryness of the mouth, unusual visual phenomena such as colors, lights, or steam, and dizziness. None of these sensations will last long or have a negative effect on the body. Continued proper practice of qigong will eventually make such sensations disappear.

BENEFITS OF QIGONG PRACTICE

There are virtually innumerable ways in which one can benefit from the practice of qigong. A deep and full rest at night is another fine condition that can be attained with the practice of qigong. Because of this practice, a person will need less sleep than usual. One will awaken a new person, replenished and ready to face a new day. After qigong practice, one will feel stronger and more energetic, and the mind will feel clear and tranquil. After prolonged training, one will feel light but strong.

The practice of qigong improves blood circulation and enriches the blood with more red blood cells. This increases the supply of oxygen to the tissues and promotes healthier tissues and organs. The greater supply of oxygen enables the heart to pump more slowly, yet still provide enough oxygen to the body. Imbalances such as high blood pressure and rapid heartbeat are made normal with prolonged, proper practice of qigong.

Qigong serves the whole body rather than one specific area, although this is possible through specific exercises. Qigong is also a way of attaining good health and peace of mind. Qigong calls on no external means, because it first of all exercises the internal organs and puts them into good running order and balance with each other. Since qigong introduces nothing into the body and depends only on the body itself to create antibodies, it is the most natural and direct method of cure.

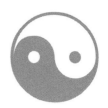

PART TWO

Hou Family Qigong

CHAPTER 3
Background of Master FaXiang Hou

Master FaXiang Hou is a fifth-generation master of qigong and has been practicing qigong as a form of exercise and as a healing art for over twenty-five years. His great-great-grandfather went to Tibet, where he studied healing arts in a Buddhist monastery for twelve years. Upon his return to China, Hou's great-great-grandfather began to use what he had learned from the Tibetan Buddhists and began practicing energy work. By their third generation of qigong heirs, the Hous had also embraced Taoism. By Zhang Hin Hou's generation, both Taoist and Buddhist principles and beliefs were equally followed by FaXiang's family, which no doubt reflected on the further application and development of their qigong form.

"We use mostly acupressure points," explains Master Hou. "Our form, loosely translated, is called 'green dragon and three special acupressure points.' That is the formal name, as we really concentrate on three special points. In Chinese it is called *ching loong san dian xue mi gong fa*. There are three secret points in the form, which make it special for us because as far as I know, only my family uses these special points."

Hou recalls his apprenticeship under his father as being somewhat unusual according to ordinary Chinese medical practices. Generally

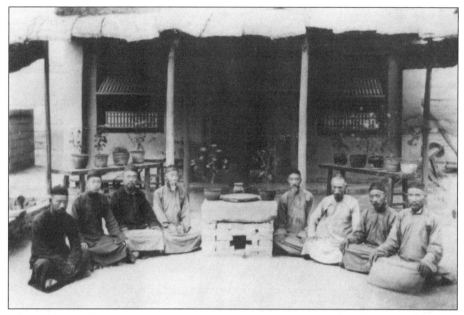

Master Hou's father and contemporary qigong masters in China.

speaking, a student of traditional Chinese medicine first learns the theory behind the system and then various methods of diagnosis. Only after years of study is one generally allowed to diagnose and then treat another person. In FaXiang's case, however, he learned specific acupuncture treatments from the onset by actually treating patients on a case-by-case basis. After becoming adept in the correct placement and number of needles needed to cure a variety of health-related problems, FaXiang was introduced to a series of qigong exercises. From these exercises, FaXiang harnessed and developed his qi, which he then used to diagnose and heal others.

Today, FaXiang Hou practices his family's form of qigong with medical applications at the forefront. Traditionally, the Hou family has been known to treat a vast array of medical problems. The specialty of FaXiang, his brother, and his father, interestingly, is working with female problems. According to Hou, they have had very good results treating female menstrual complications.

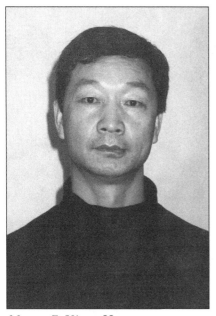

Master FaXiang Hou

Although FaXiang Hou is heir to his family's qigong legacy, he has also had the privilege of studying under four other renowned masters. In 1986, Hou learned the *san hu gong* form of qigong in San Doong Province under Master Tien Feng Kai, and is a certified teacher of that qigong form. "I practiced his form because I found it to be very simple and easy to learn," explains Hou. "I gained the energy very easily by performing the qi ball exercise."

In X'ian, Shaan Xi Province, Hou studied meditative healing exercises under a Buddhist nun named Tzu Yu, who worked mainly with deaf and mute children. The specialty of Tzu Yu is the non-touch or remote healing, whereby she is able to heal groups of people through the projection of her energy. From her, FaXiang learned how to use meditation and concentration to effect long-distance, non-touch healing.

Master Hou also studied meditation and learned various religious practices under two Buddhist monks. From studying with these men, Hou came to understand the philosophy and interrelatedness of qigong practice, Buddhism, and life through question-and-answer dialogues with the monks.

FaXiang Hou came to the United States in July of 1991 because he wanted to see the state of qigong in America firsthand. At that time he did not speak much English and needed a translator. He was eager to learn the English language because, although the level of qigong masters in China is quite advanced, they remain unable to teach many Westerners as a result of the language barrier. Hou explains that many Chinese

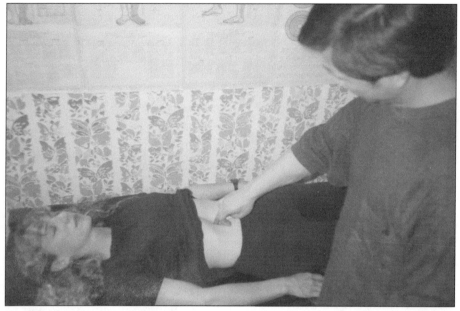

Healing a patient.

masters wish to impart their knowledge to foreigners but are unable to do so because they do not speak a second language. Master Hou found it necessary to learn English quickly since many translators did not understand the terminology that would allow them to translate his abstract concepts properly and completely to his American students.

When asked how the uninitiated could distinguish between true qigong masters and charlatans, and how his claims in particular could be supported, Master Hou retorted: "If they ask me how I learned qigong, how long I studied, and where I practiced, or any other general or specific questions about qigong, I can answer correctly. For any question you ask me I will give you an explanation. If you doubt my claims I am always willing to offer my students' names and addresses, with their approval, to contact for testimonials or recommendations. In addition, in my workshops I give an energy demonstration and teach students how to feel the qi for themselves in a very short period of time. The only way to judge the skill of a truly qualified master is by the documented results of his treatments."

And results he has, with a phenomenal success rate in healing with traditional Chinese medicine combining qigong, acupuncture, and herbology. But who could assume otherwise? After all, Hou has been recognized as a qigong master by the International Qigong Science Association, the Chinese National Qigong Association, the China Sports Qigong Research Institute, the X'ian Qigong Research Institute and Training Center, and the Healing Arts Association of San Dong, and is an instructor for the American Oriental Bodywork Therapy Association (AOBTA). No small task, given the paucity of true masters alive today, even in China.

In 1992, Master Hou founded and became director of the Qigong Research Society, an organization whose goals include introducing qigong to the general public through classes, workshops, demonstrations, lectures, books, and instructional videotapes. It is the society's goal to support clinical research of qigong and to raise public awareness of the benefits of qigong practices by presenting educational programs worldwide.

CHAPTER 4

Ching Loong San Dian
Xue Mi Gong Fa Qigong

Over the past quarter century that FaXiang Hou has been practicing, teaching, and researching his family's qigong legacy, he has developed a number of new exercises and variations on old ones. Although not necessarily bad, and definitely a matter of progression, this has led him to alter his family's form to accommodate his new outlook. "I kept my family's qigong name because the form is basically the same, I just expanded it a bit, maybe twenty-five percent. In my form, we use every movement to develop the qi. The focus is on the energy or qi in everything we do." Hou's contemporary method expresses the development of qi in three ways: slow movements, meditation, and breathing exercises.

When asked if it is possible to become sick by practicing qigong in an incorrect manner, Master Hou affirmed that nobody has ever been injured as a result of practicing his form, because he teaches students in three major steps. "The first step," states Hou, "is learning and practicing the foundation exercises, which develop a general internal energy. If you attain this internal energy, it means that you have spent a good deal of time practicing and have gotten firsthand information on how to prepare yourself and control the energy. On the second level, I teach a more specific method, where I stress correctness in movement and in thought. If you don't know the foundation and you have not yet cultivated foundation qi, you do not have anything and can hurt yourself with the later exercises. If you earnestly practice the foundation level, the secondary and upper-class levels will come easily and with no side effects."

FaXiang Hou has been teaching qigong in America for nearly a decade now. "I teach three different classes," he explains, "the foundation, continuing series, and special exercises to help teach and heal others. Within each level of qigong I introduce different meridians and their purposes. When someone graduates from my form they should know the uses of each of the meridians so that they can treat other people."

Based on the experience he has gained from teaching classes and seminars across the United States, Master Hou has found that it is generally easier for one to begin the study and practice of qigong as part of a group. "You can feel the energy much more easily and much more strongly as part of a group," Hou explains, "because everything in the world that lives has energy. The more people you have in a group, the more energy is available for the beginner to feel and experience." Hou believes that it doesn't matter if you practice qigong, yoga, or *taiji*, for they will all take time before the student is able to cultivate qi. However, Hou suggests that for those who truly wish to feel the energy quickly, his style would be a good choice. "People have felt the qi very quickly during my class or seminar. In the first hour you can feel the energy. You can later learn to use this energy to treat somebody else."

People must develop and maintain the proper qigong technique in order to protect themselves when healing others. "If you cannot protect yourself," warns Hou, "you will lose a lot of energy. The most important thing is the practice of controlling one's own energy. For example, you must understand the different uses of qigong when healing one person as opposed to doing a mass healing of over 500 people."

If the prospect of being able to heal more than one person at a time seems incredible, Master Hou offers an example. "You can heal 900 people or 9,000 people at a time if you have the proper energy and technique. For example, my third teacher, Tzu Yu, healed 500 people—all having different problems—while she was in her home. She used a method of meditative qigong healing. For bigger groups you need to combine your energy with the patients' energy. This makes it stronger, even if there are the multiple problems of headache, leg pain, back pain, and stomach pain. These are different pains, but when giving the group treatment they will be healed accordingly." Master Hou further explains that the patients will feel a sensation of warmth in their bodies, which will eventually lead to the dispersion of their pain. When attempting to heal large groups, the qigong master must use what is called the "universal energy," a mixture of energies from the healer and the universe, which, when combined, effect a positive and powerful healing energy.

From his experience with both internal and external qigong practices, FaXiang Hou has determined that the external practice is mainly for strengthening one's own body and is not generally used for healing. The external practice is used for strengthening the ligaments and muscles, but this does not imply that the practitioner has developed an internal energy. External energy is from the universe. Internal energy also helps the external by giving it more energy. "If you want to do healing you must have the internal energy," states Hou. "Although the practice differs, the internal practice and external practice help one another." Some people seem to think that the external practice is for healing. Hou will tell you that it is not, although you can use it for self-defense. Only internal energy can be used to heal yourself and others.

So, how long does it actually take for a student who is sincere and dedicated to develop qi and cultivate enough of it to be able to heal another person? Master Hou explains that roughly twelve to thirteen class-hours of diligent practice of the foundation exercises illustrated herein are sufficient for a student to really feel the qi. "Actually," he adds, "we call this step the 'first 100 days.' If you practice the foundation diligently for 100 days, you will be able to gain and maintain the qi. But, if you practice one day and not the next, although you may still feel the energy, it will not stay with you. The first 100 days is really the foundation of my qigong form."

Master Hou has developed a curriculum of qigong exercises from what he considers to be the best lessons he has learned. These exercises, along with mindful concentration and breathing techniques, are comfortable, calming, and easily performed by people of all ages and physical conditions, regardless of time or place. Whereas most qigong forms take months or even years of practice before results are noticed, Hou's form provides a rapid and strong visceral feeling of qi within a few minutes and healing results within a few hours. Moreover, after the first 100 days have passed, students can use their qi to treat themselves within three minutes of practicing the exercises.

Master Hou's ching loong san dian xue mi gong fa qigong is the only qigong form in the world that allows the practitioner to stop a patient's pain within two to three minutes, by merely touching three to five meridian points. With this in mind, Master Hou has developed applied qigong therapy programs for health professionals and bodyworkers, and a qigong healing program for the non-health-professional.

CHAPTER 5
Testimonials:
The Result of a Qigong Forum

The following are excerpts from letters Master Hou has received from patients he has treated in the United States. They are offered as a small sample of the results gained through his qigong form, ching loong san dian xue mi gong fa. "Patients of all ages and physical conditions come to my office, classes, or seminars," Hou states, "and virtually all find at least some kind of help through my qigong therapy and/or exercise."

T. P., a 60-year-old male from New Jersey, who suffered from a rare blood disorder, writes: "I was a peritoneal dialysis patient, with difficulty maintaining a safe hemoglobin level, who was receiving intermittent blood transfusions. After two qigong treatments my hemoglobin level increased from 7.6 to 9.8, accompanied by a great increase in my energy level. In addition, a right shoulder injury, which plagued me with pain since 1943, became virtually asymptomatic after two treatments with Master Hou."

S. Z., a 58-year-old female from New Jersey, who suffered constant severe back pain secondary to severe scoliosis, writes: "After many years of constant pain and increasing spinal curvature with disc degeneration, the combination of qigong treatment and exercise have made me pain free, and have actually resulted in straightening of the scoliotic curve!"

D.B., a 45-year-old female from New Jersey, writes: "I suffered from juvenile onset diabetes with multiple sequelae including diabetic retinopathy and neuropathy, fibromyalgia, and myofascial pain from adolescence through adulthood. Following twelve qigong treatments, four classes, and home practice, my back and neck are loose for the first time for as long as I can remember. My energy level has increased and I am not as fatigued. I can feel my feet with their different parts, and move my toes. My balance is improving and the diabetes seems to be under better control."

R.S., a 50-year-old female diagnosed with alopecia universalis, writes: "Over a period of three months I lost all of the hair on my arms, legs, my eyebrows, eyelashes, and most of the hair on my head. I had to wear a wig all of the time. The dermatologist gave me high doses of steroids and directed me to use various topical creams. After one month I decided to stop taking all the medicines and instead contacted Master Hou to begin qigong treatments. Within three months after my first treatment with Master Hou, my hair started growing back on my head and within the next month my eyebrows and eyelashes started growing back.

"It has been nine months since I started treatment with Master Hou and all the hair on my head has come in thick and I haven't worn a wig or hair piece in over six months."

M.G., a 54-year-old female with breast cancer, writes: "When I first met Master Hou in 1994 I was recovering from breast cancer, lumpectomy, and radiation treatment. My anxiety level was very high, my view of my health pessimistic, my energy erratic with an underlying general fatigue. I had periodic mild edema and joint pain in my arm, hip pain, knee swelling, and pain in my feet. For years I had felt 'not at home' in my own body.

"Through word of mouth, I heard about Master Hou's qigong classes. I had tried to do some qigong exercises from a book, but was unable to sustain interest. In the first semester of class with Master Hou I began to feel much more vitality, more at home in my body, and a slight lessening of my anxiety level.

"In the last three years I have practiced every day and the rewards have been enormous. Not only do I have more energy than I have since my thirties, but I have a sense of well-being that I have never before experienced. My body is free of pain, edema, and illness. My work as an artist is much more focused and pleasurable, and I have a greater sense of perspective about being a human being.

"Master Hou's teaching truly lets me experience my body and mind at its best: calm, energetic, and optimistic. He has given me a great gift that will last a lifetime."

M. M., a female recovering from a breast tumor, writes: "I took Master Hou's introductory qigong workshop four weeks after having surgery to remove a malignant tumor from my breast. The surgery had involved two separate incisions, including the removal of much lymph tissue from under my left arm. This resulted in significantly decreased range of motion in that arm as well as constant pain. By the end of the six hour workshop, the range of motion in my arm had increased to about ninety percent of normal and the pain was reduced. This was amazing considering that my doctors, as well as other breast surgery patients, had told me that it takes many months to get even near to normal range of motion.

"In addition, by the end of the workshop I was feeling more energy than I'd felt in several years. Within a few weeks I began a series of private consultations with Master Hou. I had chosen not to have radiation treatments following lumpectomy, but rather to stay healthy through nutritional and energetic therapies. I knew that mastering the flow of qi energy in my body, and relieving blockages in its flow, would be a vital part of my strategy to keep cancer from returning to my body. After each session with Master Hou, I felt more and more energy. In between the sessions, I continued doing the fundamental qigong exercises that I had learned in the workshop. My friends keep commenting about how vibrant I look. They were amazed at how quickly I recovered from a very serious health crisis. Subsequent mammograms have shown no evidence of cancer."

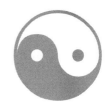

PART THREE
Building Foundation Qigong

CHAPTER 6
The Principal Qigong Points

The following points are used as a basic guide to teach beginners the Hou family qigong form. Concurrent with his mastery of qigong, Master Hou has a thorough understanding of human anatomy, and a deep knowledge of traditional Chinese medicine, including acupressure, acupuncture, and herbology. It is with this understanding that he chose these seven points to represent the principal points in his foundation course.

After a period of practice, your hands will either feel warm, swollen, or tingly. This is an indication that you have developed an awareness of your intrinsic energy, or qi. When this happens, proceed by regulating the location of main points of concentration and sensation when practicing the qigong exercises. The importance of each point is relative to the exercise you are practicing. Some will come into play more often than others. Moreover, you may feel more or less sensation at certain points, depending on the exercise at hand and the general state of health and flow of energy throughout your body. Following are the seven principal qigong points used in ching loong san dian xue mi gong fa qigong.

Principal Qigong Points

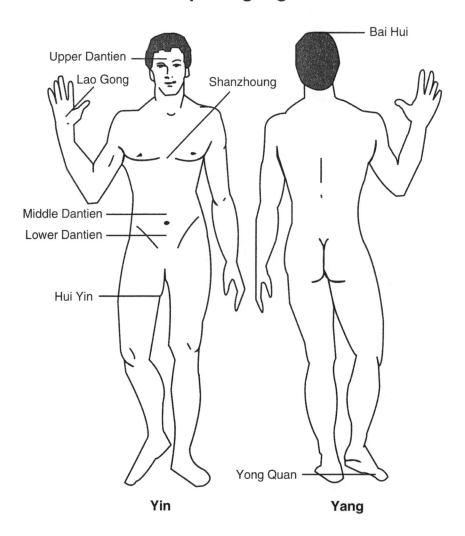

Upper Dantien

Lao Gong

Shanzhoung

Bai Hui

Middle Dantien

Lower Dantien

Hui Yin

Yong Quan

Yin

Yang

BAI HUI

This point is found at the top of the head, the location of the soft spot on a baby's head. Loosely translated, *bai hui* is the "hundred meetings" point. To locate this point, position your thumbs behind your ears, at the back of the ear lobes, and reach your middle finger to the top of your head. Where the fingers meet is the location of bai hui. As you practice qigong, you may begin to feel sensation, even soreness, at the bai hui point—this is excellent, and an indication that you are opening this important point. When the bai hui point is opened—and stays open—the practitioner can enjoy good, strong health.

UPPER DANTIAN

This point is located near the center of the forehead, both between and above the eyes. In many spiritual and healing traditions, the location of this point is referred to as the "third eye." With continued practice of the exercises outlined herein, you may feel sensation and warmth at this point.

SHANZHOUNG

This point is located in the center of the chest, between the nipples or breasts. The focus on this point should be in your chest, in general, and as though your chest were very large, like the universe.

MIDDLE DANTIAN

This point is located at the navel and surrounding area. This is the main energy center and energy storage center. Energy cultivated in the middle dantian can at once service your own body and, when properly developed, be used to help heal others.

LOWER DANTIAN

This point is located about two fingers' width below the navel, between the pubic bone and the navel. The lower dantian receives overflow qi from the middle dantian.

HUI YIN

This point is located between the genitals and anus. In Western medical terminology, this point is known as the perineum. Focus on this point and its surrounding area should be one of relaxation, because it controls the general relaxation response of the entire body.

YONG QUAN

This point is located at the ball of the foot below the so-called big toe. This is the gate of energy outflow.

LAO GONG

This point is located in the middle of the palms of the hands, or in the entire palm in general. Most qigong practitioners feel qi strongly in the hands, fingers, and palm (or *lao gong*) point.

CHAPTER 7
Fundamental Qigong Exercises

Proper and dedicated practice of the following eight fundamental qigong exercises is the key to developing foundation qi. Again, it is stressed that you should practice these exercises every day for at least 100 days. After this point, you will have developed proper qi and can then cut back on the exercises, only practicing those that you need.

Prior to beginning this set of exercises, close your eyes, relax, and clear your mind. Imagine that your head is in Heaven, that your feet are on Earth, and that you are very large, like a giant, connecting yin and yang energies. (Be sure not to imagine the Heaven and Earth connection at the beginning of each individual exercise, as this will become a distraction.)

QI BALL

The qi ball exercise teaches you how to feel, circulate, and control the flow of qi. Begin the qi ball exercise, while standing or sitting, by closing your eyes, relaxing, and clearing your mind. With your elbows bent, and your arms held away from your body, configure your arms and hands as if you were holding a basketball.

standing qi ball

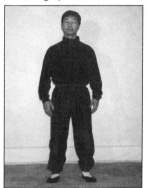 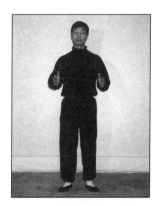 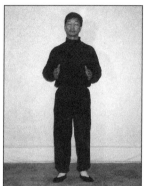

There are three ways to develop and move the energy about in your hands. The first method is to move the energy back and forth, like a ping pong ball, from hand to hand, or palm to palm.

The second method is to swirl or spin the ball in a single direction, like a globe spinning on its axis. After rotating the qi ball several times in one direction, change directions for several more revolutions. When this becomes somewhat easy, try controlling the speed at which the energy moves in each direction, alternating from fast to slow, clockwise to counterclockwise.

The third method is to hold the energy ball and begin to slowly and steadily move your hands apart and together, ever so slightly. As you pull your hands apart and then push your hands together, you may experience

seated qi ball

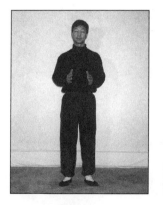 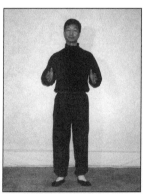 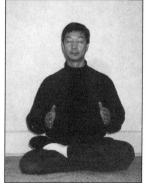

a magnetic feeling between your palms; this is the compression force of the qi. The more dense, and hence stronger, the energy, the more difficult it will be to compress it between your hands. The feeling is as if you were pushing two magnets together.

Comments: The qi ball exercise may be done formally standing or sitting as described with eyes closed, or informally while watching television, for example. This exercise may be performed for five minutes at a time or longer, as long and as often as you like. As you perform the qi ball exercise, you may begin to feel various sensations such as warmth, coolness, electricity, magnetism, and so on. All feelings and sensations are good; they are all manifestations and types of qi. Embrace them, develop them, control them.

FOUNDATION BREATHING EXERCISES

Foundation breathing exercises stretch meridians in respective areas of the body, and move qi around the organs. While doing these exercises, you may either stand, sit, or lie down. Regardless of your posture, however, it is essential that you remain loose, relaxed, and focused throughout the breaths. Breathe slowly and steadily, and physically expand and contract respective areas of the body, as dictated by the exercise.

These foundation breathing exercises have never previously been written about. They are used to treat PMS, balance hormones, treat the bowels and regulate bowel movements, treat digestive problems and regulate digestion, aid in weight control, and cleanse organs of infections and energy blockages.

To begin these breathing exercises, stand comfortably, shoulders relaxed, legs a comfortable shoulders' width apart, and with knees pointing straight ahead. Your arms should hang at your sides, and your arms,

chest breathing (front view)

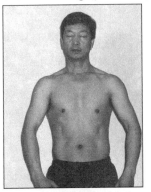 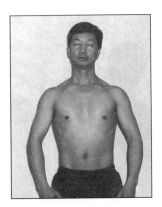

chest breathing (side view)

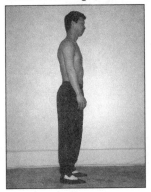 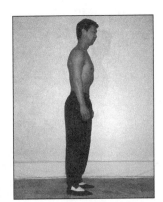

hands, and neck should be relaxed. Remember to relax the perineum (hui yin point), the point between the anus and genitals. Next, close your eyes, relax, and clear your mind.

CHEST BREATHING

The chest breathing exercise helps the respiratory system, and may be performed for five minutes at a time. Do not take big, loud, deep breaths; exhalations should last just slightly longer than inhalations.

To begin chest breathing, pull the breath and fresh energy into your lungs, by expanding them to full capacity as you inhale through your nose slowly, quietly, and steadily. Make sure to inflate the chest only. You may feel your stomach suck in slightly.

Next, as you exhale, push the breath and stale energy out through your mouth slowly, quietly, and steadily. Slowly contract your chest and lungs to their least capacity. You may feel your chest becoming concave.

UPPER STOMACH BREATHING

The upper stomach breathing exercise helps the digestive system. Do not take big, loud, deep breaths; and exhalations should last just slightly longer than inhalations.

To begin upper stomach breathing, pull the breath into the area between the navel and diaphragm as you inhale through your nose slowly, quietly, and steadily. Expand your upper stomach (only) between

upper stomach breathing

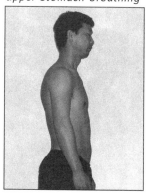 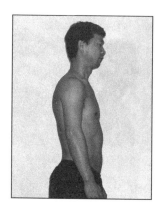 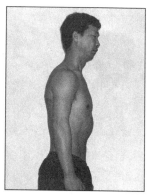

front view

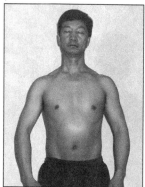 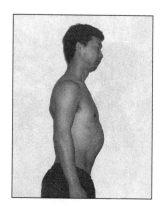

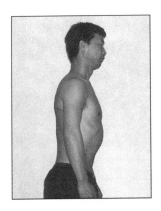 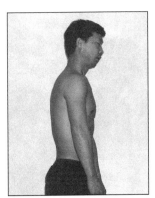

the ribcage and navel to full capacity, making sure to keep your chest and lower stomach in or flat.

Next, exhale through your mouth slowly, quietly, and steadily. Pull or suck in your upper stomach as you push your breath and stale energy out. You may feel your lower stomach pull in ever so slightly as well.

This is generally a difficult area for people to isolate in movement. Stay loose, relaxed, and focused throughout the breaths, and isolate movement only in the upper stomach.

LOWER STOMACH BREATHING

The lower stomach breathing exercise helps the reproductive and urinary systems. Do not take big, loud, deep breaths; exhalations should last just slightly longer than inhalations.

To begin lower stomach breathing, inhale through your nose slowly, quietly, and steadily. As you inhale, pull the breath into the lower stomach—only from the navel down. Expand the pelvic area, and drop the breath to the pelvic floor. As you inhale, inflate your lower stomach (only) between the ribcage and navel to full capacity, making sure to keep your chest and upper stomach flat and deflated.

Next, push the breath and stale air out, and pull or suck in your lower stomach as you exhale through your mouth slowly, quietly, and steadily. You may feel your upper stomach pull in ever so slightly.

lower stomach breathing   *front view*

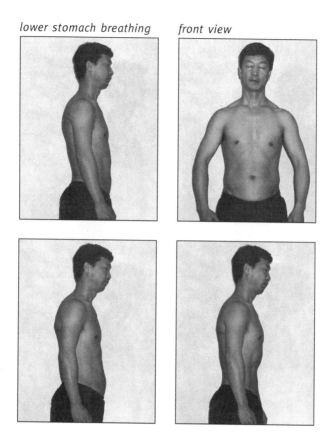

This can also be a difficult area for people to isolate in movement. Again, stay relaxed and focused throughout the breaths, and try to isolate movement in the lower stomach. With continued practice you will progress.

Comments: All three breathing exercises may either be done formally as described or informally while watching television or sitting in a bus, train, or car, for example. If done formally, men should do thirty-six breaths, while women should do twenty-four breaths, or their equivalent in time. (You should time yourself as to how long these repetitions take you to complete, and just practice for this period of time to avoid the distraction of counting repetitions.)

If done informally, there is no time or repetition limit, but do not do the exercise all day long (too much of anything is not good). Some people may experience slight discomfort when beginning these breathing exercises. This usually occurs in an area where qi is not moving freely. Continue your practice, and the discomfort will gradually cease.

STANDING POLE

The standing pole exercise aims to circulate the qi throughout the entire body and meridian system. It aids in whole-body circulation of blood and energy, utilizes the body's whole meridian system with the yin and yang forces, and stretches and adjusts nineteen vertebrae—from the coccyx to T1.

front view

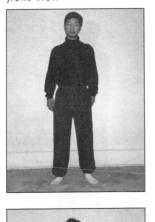
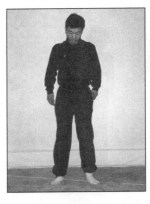
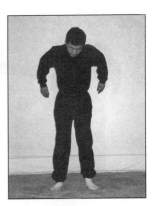
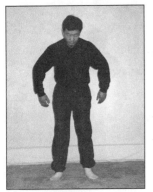
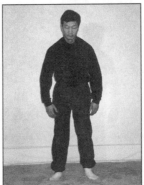
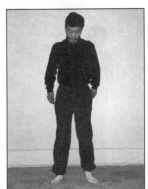

side view

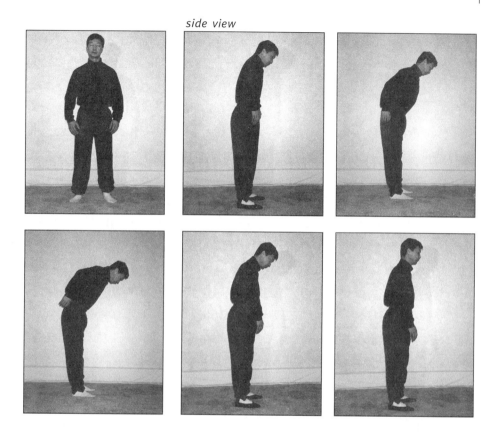

To begin the standing pole, stand comfortably with shoulders relaxed, legs a comfortable shoulders' width apart, and knees very slightly bent. Keep your arms slightly away from your torso. Your arms, hands, and neck should be relaxed. Remember to relax the perineum—the hui yin point found between the anus and genitals. Breath and movement are combined in this exercise to circulate qi throughout the meridian system. All movements should be slow, steady, and deliberate.

Next, close your eyes, take a deep breath, and clear your mind. Inhale through your nose, slowly and steadily, and bring energy up the back of your body. Exhale through your mouth, slowly and steadily, and bring the energy down the front of your body. Be sure to breathe silently and calmly, paying no attention to the sound of your breath.

With each inhalation, concentrate on pulling the qi up your back side and moving your body as the energy moves. The qi moves through your heels and up the back of your legs. As the qi passes your knees they straighten. The qi then continues past your hips up your spine to the shoulder area. When the qi reaches the base of the spine, begin to pull your shoulders up, thus moving the energy up the spine and to the top of your head (bai hui point). Your hips, waist, and spine contract and rise as the qi moves through each area.

With each exhalation, concentrate on moving the qi down your front side; the moment of moving your body should follow the energy movement. Follow the movement of qi from the bai hui point as your shoulders move forward; follow it down across your forehead and face, down your chest, and down your stomach. At this point, the qi splits off and goes down both legs as your knees bend, and out the balls of your feet (yong quan point).

Comments: Repeat this sequence for at least five minutes, but as long as you like. While performing the standing pole exercise, you should experience a feeling of warmth over each area the qi travels through. You may also experience sensations of cold or vibrations, or feel as though there is a clicking sound in your joints or spine. As your practice continues, you may feel heightened sensations in various areas of your body.

Some people may also experience slight discomfort in various areas of their body, which generally indicates a place where qi is blocked. With continued practice the discomfort will gradually cease.

THREE WHIPS

The three whips exercise teaches you how to move and store energy. It is done in a set of three (two single whips and one double whip). This exercise specifically benefits the spinal column, directly stretching from T1 to T5. In addition, it balances energy in the lungs and heart, releases stress in the neck and shoulders, and relieves related problems such as carpal tunnel syndrome.

To begin the first whip, slowly raise your left arm (for males) or right arm (for females) straight out in front of you, in line with your knee. It is essential that your hand be in line with your knee. Be sure to do this slowly and steadily, with elbow and wrist remaining straight.

first whip

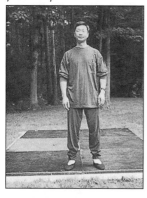
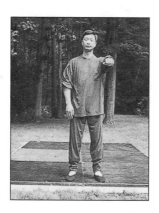
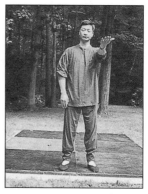
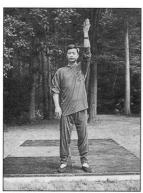
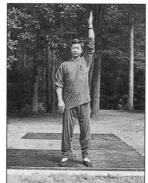
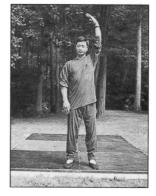

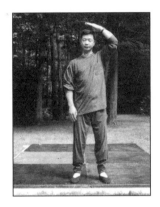 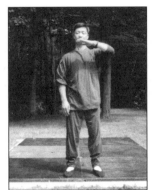 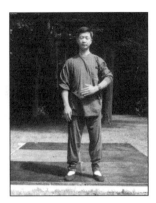

third whip

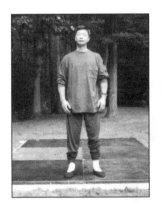 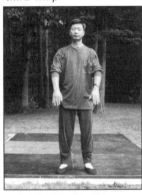 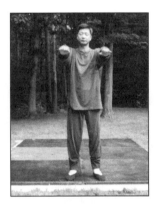

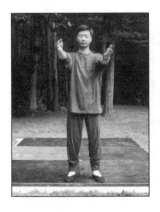 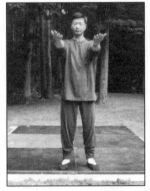 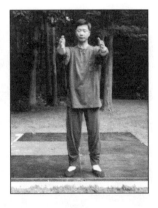

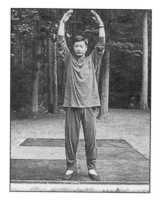
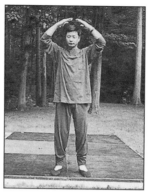
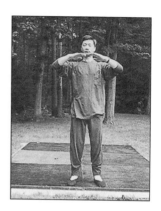

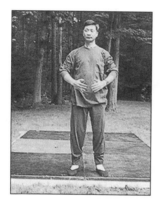
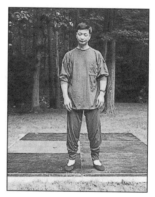

Note: You must only use your shoulder to lift your arm! As you lift your arm, your palm should face down, and you should concentrate on the idea that you are lifting the qi up from the ground. You may feel the sensation of pulling taffy.

When your arm reaches shoulder level, rotate it so that your palm faces up (again using only your shoulder). In doing this, you are mixing the yin and yang energies. You should feel a stretching across your shoulders and back. Continue to lift your arm, using only the shoulder, up above your head until your arm is parallel to your ear.

Stop briefly, and using only a flick of your wrist, drop this ball of qi onto the top of your head (bai hui point). Now, slowly push the qi into the top of your head, allowing your elbow to bend. As you move the qi to the crown of your head, tuck your thumb in slightly, preventing it from touching your face.

With your palm facing down, move the qi down your forehead, face, neck, chest, and stomach. Stop briefly at your stomach (lower dantian), to store energy there. After you feel warmth in the dantian area, let your arm return to your side. The remainder of qi will continue to travel down your legs automatically.

The second whip is performed identically to the first whip, but done with the opposite arm (right for males and left for females). Once this is done, move on to the third or double whip.

To do the third (double) whip, raise both arms at the same time (again, using only your shoulders). Maintain your arms in a straight position, and be sure to raise both arms in front of you, and in line with your knees.

When your arms reach shoulder level, rotate them (again, using only your shoulders) so that your palms face up. Then, rotate your arms half way back so that your palms face each other, as if you were holding the qi ball in your hands. If done properly, you should feel a stretching across your shoulders and back.

Next, continue to lift your arms (again, using only your shoulders), as though you were lifting the qi ball above your head, until your arms are in a straight line and parallel to your ears.

Stop briefly, and using only a flick of your wrists, drop the ball of qi onto the top of your head (bai hui point). With your palms facing down, move the qi down your forehead, face, neck, chest, and stomach. Stop briefly at your stomach (lower dantian point) to store the energy. After you feel warmth in the dantian area, let your arms return to their respective sides. The remainder of qi will continue to travel automatically down your legs.

Comments: As you lift your arms, they may either feel heavy or light. This has to do with the balance of yin and yang energy in your body, and with the time of day that you are practicing. The sensation may change from day to day, hour to hour, season to season.

As your arms move down along the front of your body, you may feel heat moving down your face, chest, and stomach, or you may feel an electric sensation on your skin, especially on the arms. In addition, you may feel qi both internally and externally, half inside and half outside of your body.

Practice this exercise nine times for each whip in any order with which you feel comfortable, but a total of twenty-seven arm lifts (or whips) is necessary.

SHOOTING SPARKS

The shooting sparks exercise aims to move qi in and out of the palms (lao gong points) while also stretching the meridians of the heals, ankles, knees, and lower back. It is important to have and maintain correct form in this exercise to truly reap its benefits. In essence, shooting sparks is the best exercise for building energy and healing injuries of the lower back, knees, and ankles, relieving neuropathy, bolstering the immune system, repairing nerve damage of the feet, and improving skin and muscle tone. Countless testimonials indicate drastic improvement from regular practice, including sixty-five percent low back improvement, eighty-five percent knee improvement, and seventy-five percent ankle improvement.

To begin shooting sparks, stand with your feet a shoulders' width apart. Your feet should be pointing forward throughout the exercise, and your heels should never leave the ground. Stay relaxed throughout your body, close your eyes, relax, and clear your mind.

front view

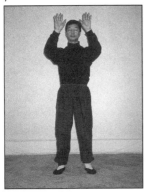 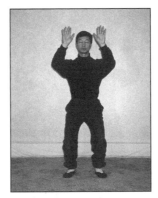 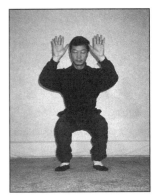

side view

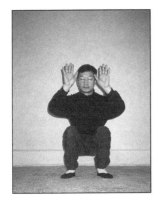 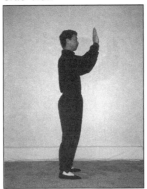 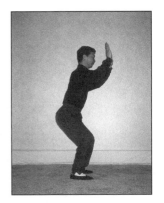

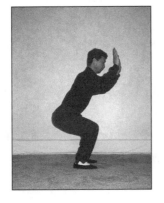 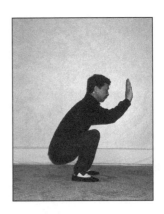

Bring your arms up to shoulder level, bend your elbows so your arms make a forty-five degree angle, and face your palms forward. Make sure your elbows are in line with your knees throughout the exercise.

Lower your body by bending your knees. As you move down to a squatting position, you should feel the qi shooting from your palms and upper dantian, like a laser beam. Exhale as you begin your descent, slowly and steadily. Move down in a straight line, keeping your back straight, and your ankles and knees should not move more than about twelve degrees.

Note: Make sure that your knees never move past the tips of your toes. In order to get into the low squat without your knees passing your toes, you may need to stick your bottom out slightly. However, it is incorrect to bend your body forward. Keep your back in a straight line at all times.

As you begin your ascent into the standing position you should feel the qi moving back into your palms (lao gong points) and upper dantian. Be sure to move into the standing position slowly and steadily, while maintaining a straight spine.

Comments: While performing this exercise, it is important that you only squat as low as you can without compromising proper form. Going too far or too fast may result in pain or injury. Patient practice of this exercise will get you completely down in a squat (correctly) in a short period of time.

Be sure to perform only nine repetitions of this exercise, and to do them correctly. During practice, you may feel a sensation of warmth come over you. This is natural.

SUN THROUGH THE POLE MEDITATION

Sun through the pole is a very simple, brief meditation that transforms external energy into internal energy.

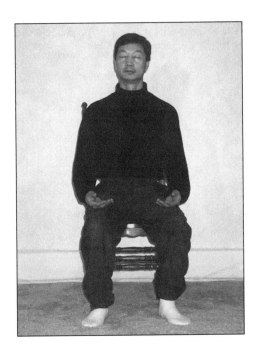

To begin the meditation, sit up straight, preferably in a full or half lotus position, with palms facing up and resting comfortably on your legs or knees. If you cannot sit in a lotus position, sit in a chair (your body should not touch the back of the chair) or on the floor with legs outstretched. Be sure to keep your back straight, and do not lean back or hunch forward. You may also lie down, but should really do so only if you find it very difficult or painful to sit straight for ten minutes.

Close your eyes, relax, and clear your mind. Imagine you are one with the universe. You are very large and simply a part of the essence that fills the universe. There is a very big, bright, hot, golden sun before you.

At the middle of your forehead (the upper dantian) there is a door. This door opens, and the sunlight and warmth come in. Then the door closes, locking in the sunlight and warmth. This sunlight and warmth move slowly down your body internally—as though traveling down a long pole through the center of your body.

First it moves down your face, then your throat and neck, then your chest, then your stomach, then to your navel (middle dantian), and below to your lower dantian.

The warmth and sunlight rest at the lower and middle dantian briefly, and then the warmth and sunlight begin to ascend. They move up through the stomach, then the chest, then the throat and neck, then up the face, and finally the door at the upper dantian opens, and the sunlight goes out.

Then, the sunlight enters in the door at the upper dantian and begins its descent again. The cycle continues as long as you feel you need.

Comments: A concentrated focus on the sun and its traveling path through the pole should be done for about ten minutes, or as long as you can keep focused. If you can not focus for ten minutes, just do it for as long as you can. Then let your mind wander in a free meditation for as long as you like. The free meditation can be any sort of place that your mind wanders—a paradise, a childhood memory, the sky, or anyplace else. Whatever you see will be clear and detailed and able to be described. However, the vision may last only three to five seconds.

CLOSING EXERCISE

The closing exercise aims to wash the meridian system, and correct energy imbalances in the body, including high blood pressure.

To begin the closing exercise, stand straight with your feet a comfortable shoulders' width apart. Stay relaxed throughout your body, close your eyes, and clear your mind.

Swiftly but not stiffly, and in a sweeping motion, raise your arms up along both sides of your body and above your head, as though you were scooping up the energy around you. (Men should raise their left hand just slightly higher above their head than their right hand. Women should raise their right hand slightly higher than their left.)

Next, softly and evenly bend at the elbows and move the palms down toward the bai hui point on top of your head, as though you were pushing energy into the point. Be sure not to touch your head.

Fold your thumbs in slightly, and move your hands down along the front of your body in a steady motion, with palms facing the ground. As your arms and hands move down, you should feel energy washing down your body, like a waterfall. The energy washes down your face, chest, and stomach, and splits off down the legs and out the balls of your feet. You may feel a rush of energy leave your feet, and you may have an external and internal sensation as the energy washes down your body.

Comments: If you have practiced qigong for fifteen minutes or more, you should end with nine repetitions of the closing exercise. As a regular exercise, this can be performed for five, ten, fifteen, or more minutes at a time.

for male

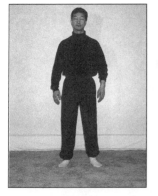
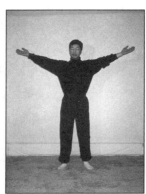
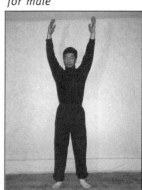

for female

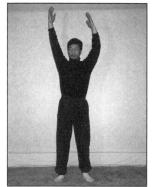 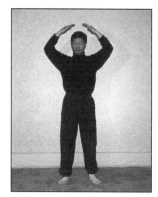 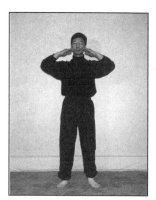

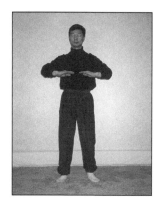 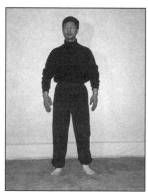

CHAPTER 8
Animal and Element Exercises

Readers wishing to move on to this next set of exercises should have already practiced the previous exercises diligently for at least 100 days. If this has not been done, the results of the following exercises will not be as profound as they could or should be. So, if you have not completed the "first 100 days," please do so before moving on.

Expertise in these exercises, as well as the sensations and energy felt while practicing, will vary from person to person, and will change as your qi develops. It is always a good idea to continue to practice and review these exercises on a regular basis.

The exercises in this section are the next step in developing foundation qigong. They include a special focus on the natural movements of animals and elements. Again, you may prefer to practice some more than others, but try to practice them all—at least as a review—so that you don't forget them. There may be times when you find you really *need* to do an exercise that you previously found undesirable.

With the addition of these seven exercises, you should have a broad base on which to begin building elementary qi within yourself. This qi should not only serve you, but may be helpful in healing others as well.

THE GOOSE

The goose exercise moves qi up and down the back and front sides of the spine, or in more technical terms, along the *ren mai* and *du mai* channels. It is also an excellent exercise for relieving tension in the back, neck, and shoulders. It helps to move stagnant energy from the chest and breast area.

To begin the goose exercise, stand straight, with your feet a comfortable shoulders' width apart. Stay relaxed throughout. Close your eyes, and clear your mind. Imagine you are a wild goose, flying gracefully through the heavens.

Next, pull your shoulders back, extending and stretching the front of your rib cage. Bend ever so slightly at the waist, just until you feel that your coccyx or lower back is carrying some weight. Bring the qi up your

front view

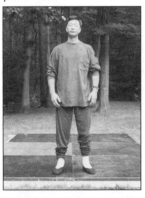
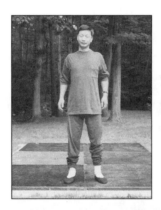
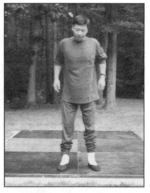
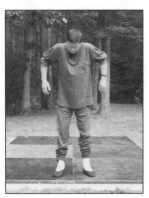
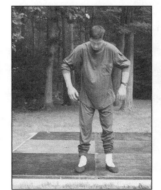
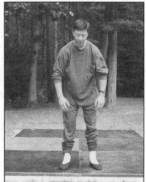

side view

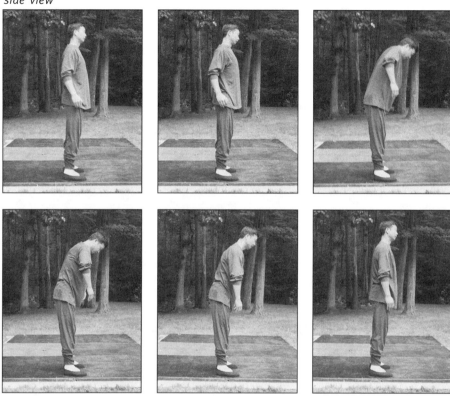

spine by rolling your shoulders up and in a half-circle forward, slowly, steadily, and without straining. Your head will naturally bend forward.

As your shoulders move forward and down, slowly raise your head. You should feel a sensation of warmth moving down your chest and the front of your body as the qi moves down your chest and breast area. Straighten your body and continuously repeat this motion slowly and flowingly. You should begin to feel a sort of progressive clicking or movement up and down each vertebra.

This exercise physically stretches the breast area and moves stagnant energy from the breast and related lymph nodes. It is useful in removing and preventing breast cysts and tumors.

Comments: The sensation of energy is more subtle in this exercise. However, as you continue to practice, the sensation of qi moving up and down the spine, vertebra by vertebra, should increase.

This exercise can be performed for five to fifteen minutes at a time or more. The areas where qi is moving during this exercise are often referred to as the "microcosmic orbit." The qi circulates in an orbit around the torso, from tail to tip and then from tip to tail of the spine.

THE TIGER

The tiger exercise moves qi up the back of the body and out through the palms (lao gong) and forehead (upper dantian).

To begin the tiger exercise, stand with your knees slightly bent and your feet a comfortable shoulders' width apart. Your hands should be flexed tightly, fingers slightly curved, held at the level of your temples. Slowly breathe in through your nose while straightening your knees, and bring the qi up the back side of your body—from the heels to your shoulders and head.

Next, quickly bend at the waist, keeping your back straight, and make your body like the shape of the number seven. This should be done

side view

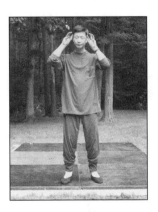
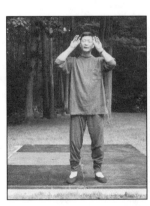

side view

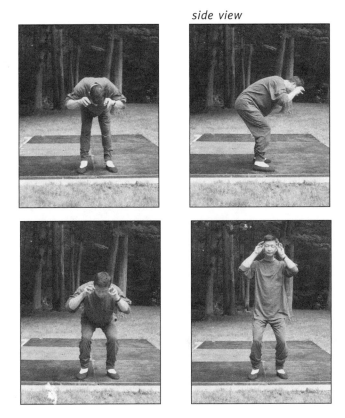

in almost a snapping motion. While bending forward, breath out quickly (but quietly) through your mouth, and shoot the energy out of your
palms (lao gong) and forehead (upper dantian).

Breathe in again, slowly rising up and straightening your knees and
back, and bring the qi up again. Bend at the waist, exhale, and release the
qi from the palms and forehead. You should repeat this sequence nine times.

Comments: Throughout this exercise your hands should never move
from the level of your temples. This is an excellent technique for relieving stale energy and learning to emit qi. If you suffer from severe or
chronic low back pain, you may want to only do this exercise three
times or you may skip it if you feel it might exacerbate your condition.

THE BEAR

The bear exercise balances your energy from side to side. Since it is a very soft movement exercise, it is important to keep every part of your body loose and relaxed throughout each movement.

To begin the bear exercise, stand with your knees loose, your feet a comfortable shoulders' width apart, and your whole body relaxed. Pick up your arms and let your hands hang loosely around your temple area—but not stiffly as in the tiger exercise. Imagine that you are a big, lumbering bear.

Slowly inhale through one nostril while bringing the qi up that same side of your body, and stretch your leg and body up as if you were taking a step. As you exhale through the same nostril, move as if you were stepping down. Your body moves forward in a loose fashion, and you should feel a

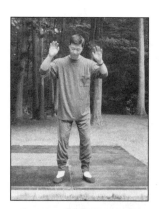
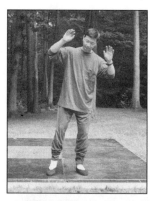
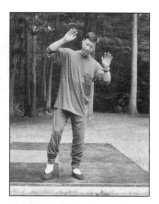
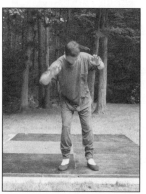
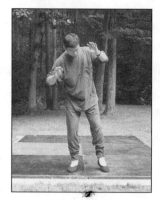
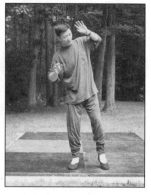

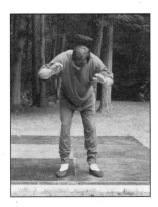 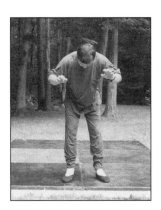

loose, soft, and flowing energy around your palm. Repeat this sequence on the opposite side, and do as many repetitions as you feel you need.

> **Comments:** You can perform this exercise "walking" or staying in the same location. This is an excellent exercise for moving qi through the nervous system, and should be practiced for five to fifteen minutes at a time, or more.

TURTLE HOLDING ITS SHELL

Turtle holding its shell is an excellent exercise for relieving tension and pain in the back, neck, and shoulders. It is helpful in correcting cervical vertebrae inconsistencies, and moves energy through the brain to help clear the mind. It is a harder (as opposed to softer) type of exercise.

To begin this exercise, stand with your feet a comfortable shoulders' width apart. Bend at the waist with your back straight, so that you are in the position of the number 7. Raise your arms up behind your back with palms facing up, as though holding a turtle's shell. Inhale through your nose, raising your shoulders up, and pulling your head in (tucking the turtle's head in) while inhaling. Remember to hold your arms up.

Next, exhale through your mouth while moving your shoulders down and stretching your neck out (sticking the turtle's head out) while

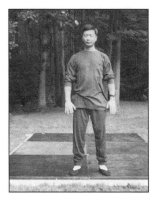
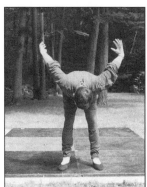

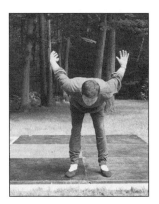
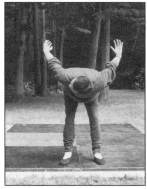

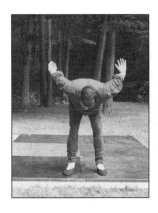
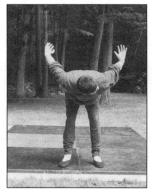
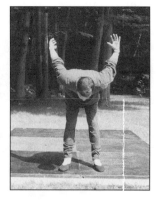

exhaling. Remember to keep your arms up. Again, inhale through your nose while raising your shoulders up, and pulling your head in. Again, exhale through your mouth while moving your shoulders down, and turning your head to the left, stretching your neck forward. Next, inhale through your nose while turning your head to the center, raising your shoulders up, and tucking your head in, and then exhale through your mouth while turning your head to the right side and out.

Comments: While performing this exercise, be sure to move slowly and steadily. Repeat this exercise to the left, right, and front an equal number of times. This exercise should be practiced correctly, nine times in each direction, in any sequence you choose. Remember to keep your arms up. Do not let them slip down as you inhale and exhale.

ROLLING PAPER

The rolling paper exercise physically stretches the spine, allowing qi to enter each vertebra as you bend forward and then straighten up. It also releases tension in the spine and the muscles running alongside it, thus providing a greater flexibility and range of motion.

front view

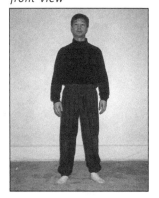 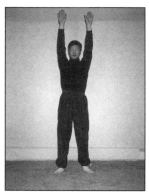 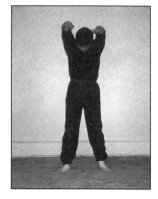

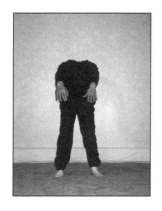
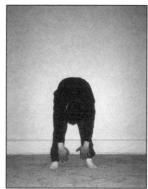
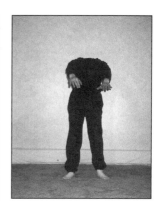

side view

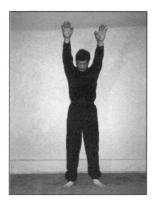
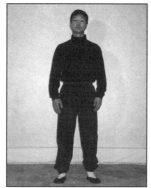
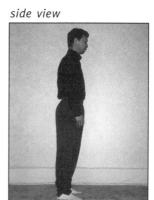

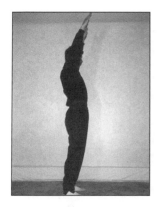
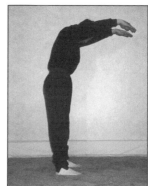
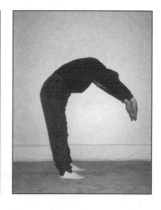

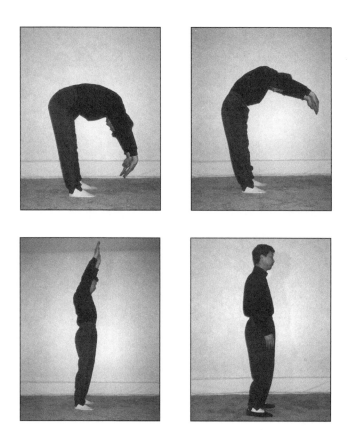

To begin the rolling paper exercise, stand comfortably with shoulders relaxed, legs a comfortable shoulders' width apart, and knees very slightly bent. Raise your arms straight up over your head, palms facing forward, until they are next to your ears.

From this position, slowly, steadily, and deliberately bend forward, stretching one vertebra at a time (from your neck to your coccyx) until you are bent fully forward and your arms touch the ground. As you bend forward, exhale naturally through your mouth. Remain in this hunched-over posture for one to two seconds before ascending, straightening your spine from coccyx to neck until your head is once again pointing up. As you rise upward, inhale through your nose.

Comments: While performing this exercise, be sure to move slowly and steadily. Breath and movement are combined to circulate qi throughout the meridian system. Be sure to keep your arms above your head and parallel to your ears throughout the exercise, which should be performed a total of nine times.

QI FROM THE ELEMENTS

The qi from the elements exercise helps to gather and store yang qi from the sun and yin qi from the moon and nature. The set of exercises, then, is divided in three: sun, moon, and nature.

Begin qi from the elements exercises by standing comfortably, with shoulders relaxed, legs a comfortable shoulders' width apart, and knees very slightly bent.

THE SUN AND THE MOON

From the beginning position, take a half-step diagonally forward with your left leg. With your eyes open, visualize that you are looking at the sun. Once you have a clear image of the sun in your mind, move your arms as if quickly embracing and picking up the sun. While doing this,

The Sun Exercise

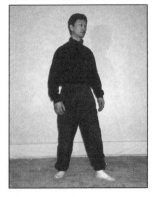 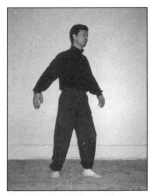 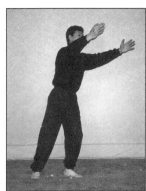

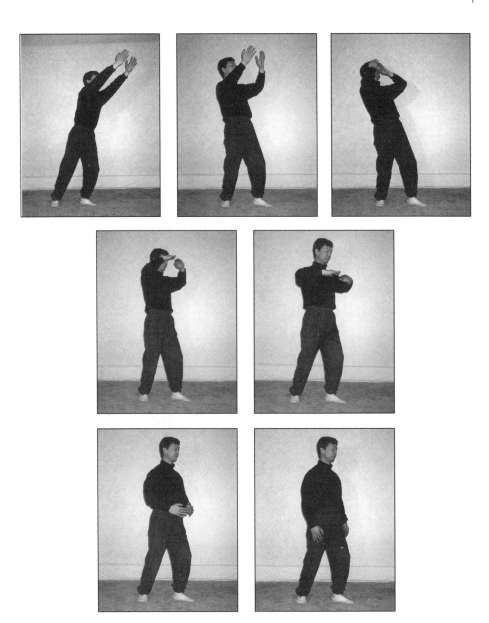

bend your front knee, but keep your back leg straight. Now close your eyes, use your front leg to shift your body backward, ending with your front leg straight and your back leg bent. As you do this, move the sun's heat energy into your upper dantian; you must pull the sun's qi into your head until your hands touch your upper dantian (mind's eye).

The Moon Exercise

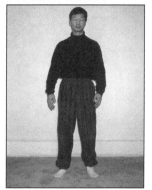
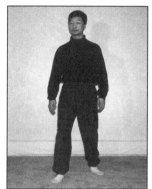
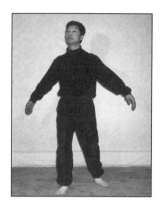

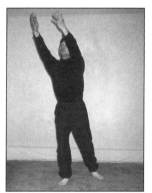
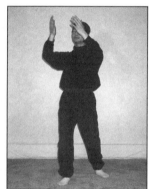
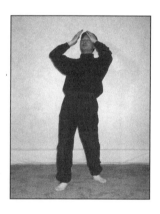

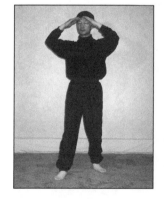
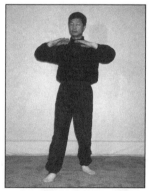

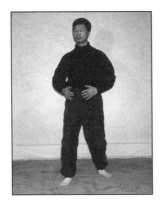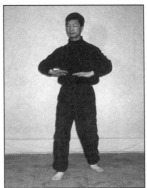

Shift your weight forward until your front knee is again bent and your back leg straight. With your palms facing down, move the qi down your forehead, face, neck, chest, and stomach. Stop briefly at your stomach (lower dantian point) to store the energy. After you feel warmth in the dantian area, let your arms return to their respective sides. The remainder of qi will continue to travel automatically down your legs.

The moon exercise is identical to the sun except that you visualize the moon and the moon's colors. In addition, since it is safe to look directly at the moon, best results are achieved if you practice this exercise while looking at the moon on the three days of the full moon.

Comments: You must do this exercise a total of eighteen times, nine times with each leg forward. While doing this exercise, you should see the colors of the sun and then of the moon in your mind's eye. Such visualization will help to manifest and spread the qi throughout your body.

NATURE

From the beginning position, take a half-step diagonally forward with your left leg. With your eyes open, visually absorb the colors of nature. You may be looking at a tree, plants, flowers, an ocean, a mountain, or all of the above. The more variety of nature that you look at and absorb, the better.

Quickly embrace and scoop up the natural environment horizontally (not diagonally upward as with the sun and moon). While doing this, bend your front knee, but keep your back leg straight. Use your front leg to shift your body backward, ending with your front leg straight and your back leg bent. As you do this, move the nature energy into your chest (between the nipples, or shanzhoung point).

Shift your weight forward until your front knee is again bent and your back leg straight. With your palms facing down, move the qi down

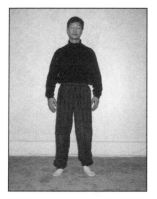
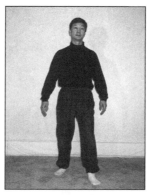
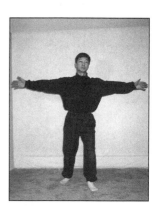
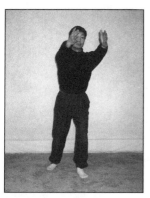
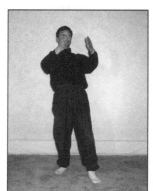
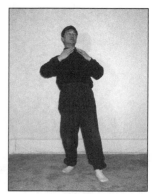

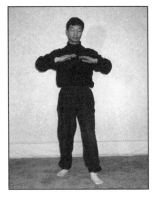
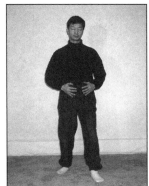
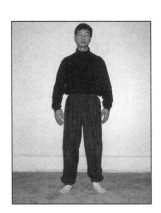

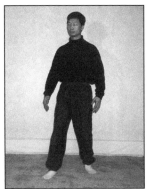
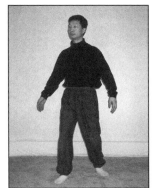
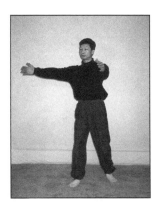

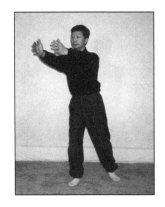
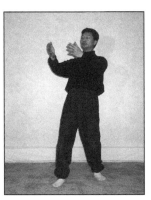

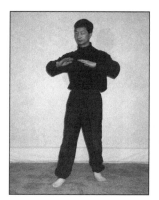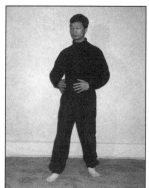

your forehead, face, neck, chest, and stomach. Stop briefly at your stomach (lower dantian point) to store the energy. After you feel warmth in the dantian area, let your arms return to their respective sides. The remainder of qi will continue to travel automatically down your legs.

Comments: Qi from the elements is an excellent exercise because it combines both the yin and yang energy from nature.

CHAPTER 9
Questions and Answers

The following are a sample of the most commonly asked questions Master Hou receives from students who attend his workshops or patients he treats. Master Hou's answers offer additional insights and supplement the information presented in Parts One and Two.

Master Hou, what is the general goal or purpose behind the practice of qigong?

People want to lead healthy, strong lives. They practice qigong because they don't want to be sick.

What is the connection between qigong and other Asian disciplines such as acupuncture, yoga, taiji, or gongfu?

Taiji, gongfu, and wushu all have qigong practice to some degree. Even yoga can be considered Indian qigong, just a different style, a different practice. You have the internal practice and the external practice. Some of the external practices, such as gongfu, stretch the external muscles. Internally, we stretch the nerves and meridians through the practice of qigong. It is just a different practice. Everybody just wants to find a way to stay healthy. These are just different ways.

Can one practice or perform qigong without first having a knowledge of meridians or acupuncture points?

Yes, absolutely.

Are there major differences in the way qigong is practiced in China as opposed to Taiwan?

I don't really know much about qigong as practiced in Taiwan. I have heard a little bit about qigong teachers in Taiwan, but about their style I am not sure. I believe that where qigong comes from makes no difference. There are many correct ways to practice it and also many wrong ways. Buddhist and Daoist methods ascribe many different names to their qigong forms, but the names don't make the difference. Some have internal components and some have external components. That is where the difference lies, if there is one.

Can qi be manifested in the body more easily through the practice of strict qigong exercises or through the study of the Chinese internal martial arts of taiji, bagua, xingyi, or liuhobafa?

Actually, proper development of qi takes a great deal of concentration and relaxation. With the practice of the Chinese martial arts, although the body seems relaxed, the mind is not really so. In gongfu, you must concentrate on the arm and foot placements, direction of energy, muscular tension, and formation of postures while moving and maintaining balance. You must also visualize their respective martial applications. It is these things that prolong the process of developing qi in the body. With so many other things to worry about, how can one concentrate solely on the internal energy? For example, there are so many thousands of martial artists practicing the Chinese martial arts, but how many of them actually have developed their qi to the level of a true master? Maybe just 100 or so. But ask them how long it took, and maybe you will not want to wait so long. But look at how many people have developed qi by merely practicing exercises of qigong. In my classes, students feel the qi in one session. Although on only a basic level, the possibilities are endless.

In its martial arts applications, is qigong used specifically to make oneself invulnerable or to limit the sensations of pain?

This is the specialty of qigong in the martial arts. You are not hurt as much by a strike from an opponent if you are strong. External injury is easy to treat. But, you may have internal injury, which is not so easy to overcome. In qigong practice you can treat people who have either an external or internal injury. Sometimes during the practice of martial arts, we inadvertently use the internal energy and hurt our partner. You must, therefore, also know how to treat and reverse these types of injuries. I frown upon those who can hurt but not heal. I like the person who, if he hurts another, he can heal them right away as well. Even if you accidentally injure yourself, you can use what is called the "emergency energy" to treat yourself. Actually, if you have strong energy you will naturally have good control. If somebody strikes you it will not hurt because you have the internal energy control—like a shield.

Is there a distinction made in the practice of qigong between hard and soft forms?

Hard practice—or gongfu—we call the external practice of qigong. Some people first practice the external and than the internal. In my style, we practice the internal first because we believe it helps the external. Some people first practice my exercises because they are very easy and simple. You can also practice to get the energy to develop the martial arts or to protect yourself. Either way, you will become very strong.

Does it take more time to develop an external (hard) or an internal (soft) qigong?

It depends on what it is that you like. Some people really like the external type of energy. But some people love the internal type. I think it depends on who is doing it and what style they like best. I know that no matter which one you practice, you will need time to build up the energy. If you want it quickly, I think that my style is very good. In my classes and workshops, people have felt the qi very quickly. In the first hour you can feel the energy, and you can then learn to use this energy to treat somebody else.

Do the internal and external qigong forms produce similar results for the practitioners?

No, not necessarily. It really depends on the kind of form you practice and what kind of use you are looking for. For example, my style is used mostly for the medical or healing purpose of treating people. Some people want to use the qi for the martial arts or fighting. Others want to demonstrate using the energy for breaking stones, and so on. It depends on what you like.

When treating a patient, are the effects of hard qigong different from those of soft qigong?

From my experience, the external practice is mainly for strengthening one's own body and is not generally used for healing. If you want to do healing you must have the internal energy. External practice is for developing strong ligaments and muscles. But external practice does not imply internal energy. External energy is from the universe. Internal also helps the external use by giving it more energy. Although the practice differs, the internal practice and external practice help one another. Some people seem to think that the external practice is for healing. It is not. You can use external energy, which comes from internal energy, for self-defense. Only internal energy can be used to heal.

Are there different meridians used in the study and practice of hard and soft qigong?

Yes, but they are very similar. In the practice of the three dantian levels, only for the middle dantian forms do we use a different point for the internal and external qigong forms. My middle dantian is located at my midsection, but some other forms' middle dantian is located at the chest. That is a difference, but nobody knows which is correct. The important thing to realize is that, regardless of the meridians used, if you want to be a healer you must cultivate the energy or qi.

In what manner does this internal qi development take place in your qigong form?

We use every movement to develop the qi. The focus is on the energy or qi in everything we do. It is developed in three ways: slow movements, meditation, and breathing exercises.

Are there any specific spiritual practices or beliefs involved in the study and development of your form of qigong?

As far as a spiritual practice, you can say yes there is, or you can say no there isn't. Saying there is may be like practicing the "magic head" exercise.

You concentrate on something and see it by using your mind to give focus. It is a concentrative practice. We want people to breathe, then become peaceful. You must try to relax. When your brain is relaxed your whole body's nerves and meridians are relaxed, so the energy can manifest itself through your body. People think this is spiritual, but for me I think it is just from the breath. But what I think is not important. If these practices help the patients and they feel the energy, that is more important than whether or not it is spiritual.

Can qigong be learned and developed personally if studied in a group class setting, or must it be learned on a one-to-one basis?

From my experience, I have found that it is generally easier for one to begin their practice of qigong as part of a group. You can feel the energy much more easily and strongly because everything in the world that lives has energy. The more people you have in a group, the more energy is available for the beginner to feel and experience.

Can qigong, when used for healing purposes, be performed on a group as a whole, or must it be individually administered?

You can heal an unlimited number of people at one time if you have the proper energy and technique. For example, my third teacher, Tzu Yu, healed 500 people with different problems while she was at home. She used a method of meditative qigong healing. For bigger groups you need to use your energy with the patients' energy, which makes it even stronger. Even if there are the multiple problems of headache, leg pain, back pain, and stomach pain. These are different pains, but when giving the group treatment they will all be healed accordingly. The patients will feel a sensation of warmth, which will lead to the removal of their pain.

For large groups, the healer uses what is called "universal energy." The energy of the healer, the patients, and the universe are all mixed and hence changed. Any problem can be treated this way.

Is qigong practiced differently for males and females?

They are the same. Actually, when I treat patients I am not considering whether they are male or female. Each person has different energy.

When attempting to use qigong to heal an individual with a liver problem induced from excessive alcohol consumption, would the specific treatments be different than, say, for someone who was experiencing cancer?

I think this question is really a medical question. In Eastern medicine they don't distinguish whether you are sick from alcohol or cancer. Rather, they believe that it is your meridian that has a problem. For example, if you drink excessively you will experience a liver problem. The liver helps make the blood. People need blood every moment, and so we treat any disease or virus by meridians. Your body's meridians have the problems. Determining which meridian needs healing depends on the patient's specific problem. For example, a liver problem can begin in the liver, or other organs can have a problem which has affected the liver. A healer must determine where the root of the problem is. Experience tells you what and where the root of the problem is. The qigong healer can then help the patient's liver energy balance. If the kidney energy is bad, the color of the urine will change. In Eastern medicine we have different methods of diagnosing what type of problem a patient has, such as taking the pulses, smelling the breath, or observing the skin's color. All this information can lead you to know what the patient's true problem is.

If you are using qigong to heal somebody, is there a chance that the patient may be injured if he or she has never experienced the transfer of qi from another person before?

I have never experienced this problem with my students. But, I have heard of some qigong forms that have negative side effects when the wrong treatment is performed. In fact, some people have gone crazy. However, I can guarantee that my qigong form has no side effects. My qigong form is now practiced by almost 10,000 people, and to date no one has been hurt on any level.

Could people injure themselves by developing a bad or negative qi incidental to practicing improper or unsupervised qigong?

Under my tutelage, no, because I teach in three major steps. The first step is the foundation exercise, which helps build the general internal energy. If you have this energy that means you have spent a lot of time practicing and have experienced firsthand how to prepare yourself and control the energy. On the second level, I teach a more specific method where I stress correctness in movement and in thought. If you don't know the foundation thoroughly, you have not cultivated the energy and experience and can hurt yourself with the later exercises. If you earnestly practice the foundation level, the secondary and upper-class levels will come easily and with no side effects.

I can only wonder if you have come across many individuals who have laid claim to being masters of qigong, when, in fact, they were no more than frauds?

I think America has this problem because qigong is a new phenomenon here and people want to learn it. These people, even if they practiced for a long time by means of books or videos, still have the problem of not having spent enough time under a qualified master. They may feel and really believe that they have the energy. But if you want to start teaching people, you have to completely know the form you are teaching. I don't mind people who want to teach the beginning, if they thoroughly know the beginning. They just shouldn't claim that they are masters. Beginning means you don't have the experience. The more you practice and teach, the more experience you have.

How does the aspiring qigong student determine who, in fact, is a legitimate master?

There are some specific questions that can be asked. A lot of people want to learn qigong, martial arts, or taiji. It is very difficult for them to find a good teacher themselves. A lot of people I know have come to my class only a few times and have already begun to teach qigong at their school. I cannot say that these people are not learning my form, but these people don't have the right experience. This is a very hard question you ask me because I think people should learn a qigong system under an experienced master. If you want to learn qigong or martial arts, I welcome you as my student. But if you want to open a school, you must have lessons first. I teach my students well, and if they pass the three levels I will certify them and they can teach.

How does a student of qigong determine when he has developed an adequate level of qi in his body?

In my practice, I always help students to build up the qi energy and to be able to feel the increasing levels of qi in their body. In addition, I frequently encourage my students to take the opportunity to heal patients, and ask for my guidance. You will know your level of qi development right away by your ability or inability to heal patients. You know how many patients you have treated and what the end results are. That is the test.

How does a qigong master determine when a student has developed a substantial enough level of qi to be given permission to go out and teach or heal others?

I can feel the level of qi that resides in my students' bodies. I teach people that although they may have developed the necessary energy to be able to teach another, they must first learn the method of imparting the lessons of qigong. They must have the proper teaching techniques in order to protect themselves. If you cannot protect yourself you will lose lots of energy. The most important thing is the practice of controlling one's own energy. For example, you must understand the different uses of qigong when healing one person as opposed to doing a mass healing of over 500 people.

For those who have dedicated themselves to the study of your qigong form, what is the average time it would take them to experience a "grand circulation" of qi in their body?

Roughly twelve or thirteen class-hours of dedicated learning and practice of the foundation forms is sufficient. After this amount of time, people have been known to really feel the qi in their bodies. Actually, we call the first step the "first 100 days." If you practice the foundation diligently for 100 days you will be able to gain and maintain the qi. However, if you practice one day and not the next, although you may still feel the energy, it will not stay with you. The "first 100 days" is really the foundation.

I teach my classes once a week for one hour. So, each month is four hours, with twelve hours being the basic course. I don't have the time control. If the student practices more, he or she will experience more results. After these three months you will be able to maintain the energy and actually use it to treat people on a basic level.

Is the study of alchemy or herbology separate from or a part of the practice of qigong?

These are different practices. I also practice herbal medicine and acupuncture, but the qigong exercise and healing is another form altogether. I do, however, often use them together when healing patients. But in America I do not use acupuncture because I do not yet have the license for acupuncture in the United States, only in China.

I should mention that those who graduate from my qigong form will know the Eastern medical theory of whole-body treatments. Within each level of qigong, I introduce different meridians and their purposes. When you graduate from my system, you should know the uses of each of the meridians so that you can treat people.

In China, are there governing bodies or institutions that certify and regulate the skill level of qigong practitioners and/or masters?

In China, qigong dates back over 3,000 years. The different generations in China have had their own share of politics but not a very good control of each style or form. Qigong masters in China have only been registered and certified since 1986. Actually, in 1970, China first used qigong treatments to help their Olympic teams. They had very good results. They later formed organizations utilizing people who practice in the temples and have developed a high level of qi. These people were then given certificates after being put through a rigorous test of healing.

What have you done to perpetuate qigong in America?

Well, I came to the United States in July of 1991 because I wanted to see first-hand what the level of qigong was in America. I came here to live in Shelly Fleischman's home because she was my first patient in New Jersey. I first treated her for migraines. Later I treated her for broken bones and torn ligaments due to a skiing accident in Canada. The doctor wanted her to have surgery, but I said that I could give her treatments. She is now recovered 100 percent! Another girl that I treated for a smaller condition was able to remove her crutches in six weeks. Another Chinese medical doctor helped me with translations in the beginning. She also believes that we need to help the American people and give them the opportunity to learn about authentic qigong. So, together we founded the Qigong Research Society, and although we are still in our developmental stage, we are developing a strong group of dedicated students.

How can people who are interested learn more about qigong and the Qigong Research Society?

Those who are interested can send us a letter or call us. But, I don't want students to contact us unless they desire to study with me seriously. They must pass the foundation practice. If people can pass the foundation, I will teach the advanced material. These people can eventually go on to use qigong for healing purposes if they stay true to their study. If people just want to come to my class because they want to see a demonstration and witness magic—I am not interested in that. I am looking for the more serious students who wish to help themselves first and then go on to help others.

Are there any last comments you would like to make concerning the current state of qigong?

I really hope that this book is able to help the American people to know what qigong energy is. I think that in this country a lot of people who need help do not know how or where they can find it. I hope this book is able to direct the people to a competent qigong master, or Eastern healer, and inspire in them a new interest.

Afterword

 I hope that the exercises presented in this basic instructional manual serve you well in restoring and maintaining your health and well-being. The art of qigong, while centuries old, is as current in our modern society as it is timeless.

Although no single text alone can substitute for the one-on-one instruction of a competent master, perhaps this book can put you on the right path toward finding one and give you a foundation from which to build. In my seminars I frequently tell my students that initially they must be selfish. They must think only in terms of themselves when learning and building foundation qigong. The participants are often shocked by this statement and reply that being selfish is not acceptable and that they are learning qigong not only to heal themselves, but to help others as well. To this, I say that if you cannot first help yourself, how can you expect to help another? You must be selfish in your thirst for knowledge and mastery of the foundation exercises presented herein; only then will you gain and maintain the proper qi. Once this has been achieved, you will be able to use your energy and skills to heal others. You must dedicate your time and energy to the proper practice and perfection of qigong for at least 100 days. Only then can a foundation be built.

During the course of your qigong practice, you may have questions about what you have learned or comments, about the results you may experience. Please feel free to contact me at the Qigong Research Society with your questions and comments and I will try to offer helpful advice. You may also contact me if you wish to attend one of my workshops or lectures, or receive a private healing. I am always happy to help the sincere qigong enthusiast and offer my services when available.

I wish you luck on your pursuit toward health and well-being.

—Master FaXiang Hou

Qigong Research Society
3804 Church Road
Mt. Laurel, NJ 08054
U.S.A.

Glossary

BAI HUI: This point is found at the top of the head, the location of the soft spot on a baby's head. Loosely translated, bai hui is the "hundred meetings" point.

CHING LOONG SAN DIAN XUE MI GONG FA: Literally translated as "green dragon and three special acupressure points," this is the qigong form of the Hou family. FaXiang Hou is the fifth-generation master of this form, which expresses the development of qi in three ways: slow movements, meditation, and breathing exercises.

DANTIAN: The so-called "field of elixir" where qi is gathered and stored. There are three dantians identified in the qigong system presented in this book: lower, middle, and upper.

DU MAI: Specific meridian or energy channels that run along the back of the spine.

HUI YIN: This point is located between the genitals and anus, and controls the general relaxation response of the entire body.

LAO GONG: This point is located in the middle of the palms of the hands, or the entire palm in general, and is where many practitioners feel qi the most strongly.

QI: The psychophysical principle of traditional Chinese medicine consists in the belief that a latent intrinsic energy known as qi permeates the body. It is the relationship between the intrinsic energy and the gross physical body that determines the degree to which illness or health prevails.

QIGONG: Ancient Chinese health exercises for regulating the body, the mind, and the breath that involve movement and self-massage to effect changes in health. More specifically, qigong is the art of exercising the jing (essence), qi (vital energy), and shen (spirit), the goal of which is to circulate, build, and balance qi throughout the body to promote physical and mental well-being.

QIGONG RESEARCH SOCIETY: In 1992, Master Hou founded and became director of the Qigong Research Society, an organization whose goals include introducing qigong to the general public through classes, work-shops, demonstrations, lectures, books, and instructional videotapes. It is the society's goal to support clinical research of qigong and to raise public awareness of the benefits of qigong practices by presenting educational programs worldwide.

REN MAI: Specific meridian or energy channels that run along the front of the spine.

SAN HU GONG: The qigong form of Master Tien Feng Kai from San Doong Province, China.

SHANZHOUNG: The point located in the center of the chest, between the nipples.

YIN/YANG: A set of terms commonly used to describe various opposing physical conditions of the body. Yang corresponds to what is masculine, active, creative, bright, and hard. Yin is the feminine, passive, receptive, dark, and soft. As these concepts are applied to medical analysis of the human body, yin refers to the tissues of the organ, while yang refers to its activity.

YONG QUAN: The point that is located at the ball of the foot below the big toe, and is the gate of energy outflow.

Further Reading

Beinfeld, H. & Korngold, E. (1991). *Between Heaven and Earth: A Guide to Chinese Medicine.* New York: Ballantine Books.

Chen, C. C. (1989). *Medicine in Rural China: A Personal Account.* Berkeley: University of California Press.

Cohen, Kenneth S. (1997). *The Way of Qigong: The Art and Science of Chinese Energy Healing.* New York: Ballantine Books.

Dong, P. & Esser, A. H. (1990). *Chi Gong: The Ancient Chinese Way to Health.* New York: Marlowe & Company.

Eisenberg, David. (1987). *Encounters with Qi: Exploring Chinese Medicine.* New York: W. W. Norton & Co.

Hou, FaXiang & Wiley, Mark V. (1998, April). Qigong in the Martial Arts. *Martial Arts Legends*, pp. 58–66.

Kaptchuk, Ted J. (1983). *The Web That Has No Weaver: Understanding Chinese Medicine.* Chicago: Congdon and Weed Publishers.

Lehmann, A. C. & Myers, J. E. (1989). *Magic, Witchcraft, and Religion*. Mountain View, CA: Mayfield Publishing.

Major, J. S. (1987a). Ch'i. In M. Eliade (Ed.), *The Encyclopedia of Religion* (Vol. 3, pp. 238–39). New York: Macmillan.

Major, J. S. (1987b). Yin-yang Wu-hsing. In M. Eliade (Ed.), *The Encyclopedia of Religion* (Vol. 15, pp. 515–16). New York: Macmillan.

MacRitchie, J. (1993). *Chi Kung: Cultivating Personal Energy*. Boston: Element Books.

Maliszewski, Michael. (1992). Medical, Healing, and Spiritual Components of Asian Martial Arts. *Journal of Asian Martial Arts, 1* (2), 24–57.

Reid, Daniel. (1995). *The Complete Book of Chinese Health and Healing*. Boston: Shambhala.

Shih, T. K. (1994). Disease and Senility: Two Enemies of Longevity. *Qi: The Journal of Traditional Eastern Health and Fitness, 4* (1), 24–31.

Shih, T. K. (1994). Qigong Elicits Latent Energy and Promotes Intelligence (part two). Qi: *The Journal of Traditional Eastern Health and Fitness, 4* (3), 10–13.

Shih, T. K. (1994). *Qigong Therapy, the Art of Healing with Energy*. Barrytown, NY: Station Hill Press.

Veith, I. (1972). *The Yellow Emperor's Classic of Internal Medicine*. Berkeley: University of California Press.

Wiley, Mark V. (1995). An Interview with Hou FaXiang Concerning Qigong Practice. *Journal of Asian Martial Arts, 4* (3) 61–75.

Wiley, Mark V. (1996). The Healing Ways of FaXiang Hou. *Qi Gung Kung Fu*, pp. 52–56.

Wong, Kiew Kit. (1993). *The Art of Chi Kung: Making the Most of Your Vital Energy*. Boston: Element Books.

Yang, Jwing Ming. (1991). *The Root of Chinese Chi Kung*. Jamaica Plain, MA: YMAA Publications.

Yun, G. (1990). *Qigong for Life*. Cosmax International.

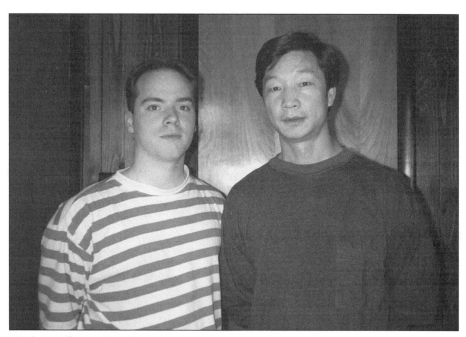

Mark V. Wiley and FaXiang Hou

About the Authors

FaXiang Hou is the fifth-generation heir to his family form or qigong, known as ching loong san dian xue mi gong fa. It is a unique form of medical qigong which focuses on the use of three special acupressure points when healing a patient, in addition to self-practice exercises. Hou is recognized as a qigong master of several of the leading organizations in China and immigrated to the United States in 1991. In 1992, he founded the Qigong Research Society in Mt. Laurel, New Jersey, where he resides and treats patients full time.

Mark V. Wiley has been practicing various forms of qigong in the United States and Asia for over a decade, and is a student and patient of FaXiang Hou. In addition to his interest in qigong, Mark has researched and studied traditional healing arts in the Philippines, Malaysia, Tawian, and Japan.